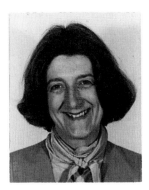

Rowan Hillson, MD, MRCP is a Consultant Physician with a special interest in Diabetes at The Hillingdon Hospital, Middlesex. She wrote her first books about diabetes while working in Oxford where she completed several diabetes research projects. Now she shares the care of several thousand people with diabetes with other members of the Hillingdon Diabetes Team. Dr Hillson is an enthusiast of outdoor activities and several times a year she takes groups of people with diabetes on Outward Bound courses. She works closely with the British Diabetic Association, and has a particular interest in helping people with diabetes to learn more about their condition.

DIABETES:
A BEYOND BASICS GUIDE

Rowan Hillson, MD, MRCP

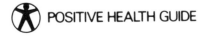 POSITIVE HEALTH GUIDE

This book is for Catherine, Michael, Anne, Sharon, Tracy, Robert, Neil, Patrick, Tula, Peter, Suzanne, Georgina and the four Pauls – people with diabetes who had the courage to have a go – and for the others who have followed them at Eskdale.

© Rowan Hillson 1987

First published by Macdonald Optima in 1987

This revised edition published in 1992

British Library Cataloguing in Publication Data

Hillson, Rowan
　　Diabetes: a beyond basics guide. –
　　(Positive health guide)
　　1. Diabetes – Handbooks, manuals, etc.
　　I. Title　　II. Series
　　362.1'96462　　RC660

　　ISBN 0 356 20564 9

Optima
A Division of
Little, Brown and Company (UK) Limited
165 Great Dover St
London
SE1 4YA

Phototypeset by BookEns, Saffron Walden, Essex
Printed and bound in Great Britain by
BPCC Hazells Ltd
Member of BPCC Ltd

Contents

Acknowledgments

I wish to thank all my friends and patients who have diabetes for teaching me about their condition. Without them this book would never have been written. I am especially grateful to those who have participated in the BDA/ Outward Bound Mountain Courses over the years. I am also grateful to my parents, my brother Simon and my colleagues at the Radcliffe Infirmary for their encouragement. Considerable thanks are due to Ms Mary Banks, Mr and Mrs W. R. Hillson, Dr Derek Hockaday, Dr Jim Mann, Mr Roger Putnam and Dr Nicholas Rose for reading the manuscript drafts and for their very helpful suggestions and continued support.

I would also like to thank Mr Jerry Bennett and his fellow instructors at the Outward Bound Mountain School, Eskdale; Mr Kevin Brown, Ms Penny Earle, Ms Edwina Armitage and the British Diabetic Association; my medical, nursing and dietetic colleagues who have helped with the BDA/Outward Bound Courses; and Oxford Regional Health Authority.

1987   RMH

The publishers would like to thank the following for their help in the preparation of this book:

For permission to reproduce the photographs: Diabetic Care Ltd, Malvern Wells, Worcestershire (pages 46 and 111); Nordisk-UK, Epsom Downs, Surrey (page 36, *below*).

For permission to reproduce the insulin list on page 27, MIMS December 1991 (this diagram is updated in each month's issue of MIMS).

We would also like to thank Dr R. Holman, Diabetes Research Laboratories, Radcliffe Infirmary, Oxford for the source of the diagram on page 22.

We thank Philip Dove, Director, Department of Medical Illustration for his assistance.

The photographs on pages 17, 28, 34, 45, 68, 83, 116, 123 and 135 were taken by David Floyd and Nick White at the Department of Medical Illustration, John Radcliffe Hospital, Oxford. The modelling was by Sally-Ann Gaul.

The diagrams are by Kevin Marks.

Introduction

Hundreds of thousands of people have diabetes. They are people in all walks of life, of all ages, and you. When your diabetes was diagnosed the doctor probably told you that diabetes is a condition in which the pancreas stops making enough insulin to allow the body to use up all the glucose derived from starchy and sugary carbohydrate food. The glucose builds up in the blood stream until it overflows into the urine where it can be detected and diabetes diagnosed. Your doctor then told you that you had to follow a special diet and take pills or insulin regularly. He told you to test your blood or urine at specific times and write down the results. That is all that many people with diabetes do to control it. They think that it is their doctor's job to make adjustments to treatment, and not their own responsibility. They feel that something terrible will happen if they interfere with the management of their own diabetes. But whose diabetes is it, yours or the doctor's?

Of course, everyone needs the simple explanation given above, but why leave it at that? You are the person who has to live with your diabetes all day, every day. *You* should be the person who knows most about your diabetes. Your diabetic advisory team of doctor, nurse, dietitian and chiropodist are all there to help you. Gradually, more and more diabetics are taking responsibility for their own diabetes and altering their treatment according to their own blood glucose measurements and what they are planning to do. Gradually, the old idea of diabetes as a disability is disappearing. I believe that with common sense and careful preparation, people with diabetes can do virtually everything they want to do. Your diabetes should not stop you from enjoying life in the way you choose. **You command your diabetes, it does not command you.**

There are many excellent books for beginners in the diabetic world. This book is not for beginners. It is for people who have already grasped the basic principles and who want to learn more about their diabetes and how to command it. I think of you, my reader, as a lively, go-ahead person, already well-informed about many aspects of your diabetes. You want to live life to the full, without your diabetes getting in your way, but without losing control of your blood glucose or increasing your risk of tissue damage.

There are different types of diabetes. You may have insulin-dependent diabetes – your pancreas is incapable of producing insulin and you would develop ketosis and rapidly become very ill without insulin injections. You have non-insulin-dependent diabetes – your pancreas is producing some insulin but you require the help of a diet and possibly the addition of oral hypoglycaemic pills. Those with non-insulin-dependent diabetes are less likely to develop ketones than insulin-dependent people. You may have diabetes associated with another hormone condition or hormone treatment (for example, steroid drugs).

Types of treatment vary also: insulin and diet, oral hypoglycaemic pills and diet, or diet alone. You may have been told that you have 'mild' diabetes or 'severe' diabetes. I do not use these descriptions because everyone with diabetes can be at risk of developing tissue damage whether they need insulin injections or diet alone to treat their diabetes. Whatever kind of diabetes you have, and however it is treated, it is important to find out precisely what is happening to your body, to learn as much as you can about your diabetes, and then to find out what is available to help you to look after yourself as well as you possibly can.

In the book I refer to doctors as 'he' and nurses or dietitians as 'she'. This is to avoid saying 'he/she' all the time – but of course health care professionals may be male or female. Throughout the book I use the proper names for parts of the body or conditions, but they are all explained in the text and there is a glossary at the end. It is important that you understand medical terminology so you can communicate well with your doctor.

This book represents one doctor's suggestions of ways of coping with different problems. Remember, there may be several ways of dealing with a particular situation and that what is appropriate for one person may not suit another. If you are not sure about any of the suggestions in this book, please discuss them with your own doctor.

Introduction to second edition

In re-reading *Diabetes: A beyond basics guide* I found it hard to remember how revolutionary the book was when it was first published. It arose out of a brief conversation with an editor, Mary Banks, who was visiting me about illustrations for another book. I said that I thought it was time someone realised that people with diabetes wanted to know more than just the basic knowledge they were usually taught. They wanted to know enough to be able to take full control of their diabetes and to make optimal use of professional help. A little later (and somewhat to my surprise) Mary Banks and Martin Dunitz contacted me and invited me to write the book. In 1987 it was considered unusual to provide people with diabetes with such detailed information. But if you are to care for your diabetes yourself, you need detailed information to enable you to assess what is happening and to take necessary action. The fact that the British Diabetic Association receives approximately 80,000 calls a year asking questions about diabetes indicates the thirst for knowledge among those who have the condition and their families and friends. Diabetes care has moved a long way since the discovery of insulin 70 years ago and continues to move forward. There have been many changes since the first edition of Beyond Basics was published. In the UK disposable syringes and needles and blood glucose testing strips are now available on the NHS and insulin injections pens are free – previously patients had to buy all of these. The St Vincent Declaration and the European Patients' Charter (see *Diabetes: A New Guide*) have been published recently establishing goals for diabetes care.

Since writing *Diabetes a Beyond Basics Guide* I have had letters from all over the world for which I would like to thank the writers. Some of them have been very informative and some very kind. Some have nearly broken my heart. It is clear that some people with diabetes, both at home and abroad, have failed to obtain the basics of diabetes education for self-care – and desperately want it. There may be many reasons for this – in some countries all health care resources are limited, in many the provision of specialist diabetes care from doctors, nurses, dietitians and chiropodists is patchily distributed about the country. In some instances, people may slip through the diabetes education net in a specialist centre. And all of us, people with diabetes and diabetes care professionals alike, need revision sessions. To help ensure appropriate provision of diabetes education, join your local or national diabetes association. The International Diabetes Federation will provide the address (page 165). Your support will help others.

Diabetes: a Beyond Basics Guide is not a basic diabetes text. It is written for people who already know something about their diabetes but want to know more. For basic knowledge read *Diabetes: A New Guide*, *Diabetes Beyond 40* or *Diabetes: A Young Persons' Guide*.

Discussions I have had with people with diabetes has suggested that some of them feel shy about asking their own doctors and diabetes team members questions. Don't be shy. That is what they are there for. Please remember that this book is a general guide to some aspects of diabetes and that you and your diabetes doctor and his or her team need to work together on your individual diabetes care. Never be afraid to ask for help.

1 Taking command of your diabetes: finding out what is happening

To take command of your diabetes you need to know what is happening in your body. To do this, you need to know what resources are available to help you to gather this information and to use it to manage your diabetes.

What information do I need?

The effects of diabetes upon the body can be divided into biochemical and physical factors. The lack of insulin or its failure to act properly at the surface of the body's cells leads to many changes in body chemistry. The most obvious, and in practical terms the most important, is an accumulation of glucose in the blood stream because it cannot enter the cells. High blood glucose levels may cause immediate symptoms (for example, thirst and passing urine frequently). In combination with other as yet unidentified factors, they may cause longterm physical damage to body tissues. You therefore need to know:

1. What your blood glucose level is
2. What effect (if any) the diabetes is having on your body over the years. This is discussed in Chapter 4.

Blood glucose monitoring

Diagnosing diabetes

Before considering what your blood glucose level is, it is important for you to know what the numbers mean. What glucose level, for example, means that you have diabetes? What level is undeniably in the non-diabetic range? This distinction has occupied many committees for many years. The World Health Organisation has produced the most widely agreed guidelines.

The diagnosis of diabetes must be made before any treatment is begun. The internationally agreed guidelines assume that people are eating their usual diet and not taking glucose-lowering medication. If you have symptoms of diabetes (for example, thirst and passing a lot of urine), a single laboratory measurement of glucose in a sample of blood taken from a vein is sufficient to make the diagnosis of diabetes. If the glucose concentration is 7.8 mmol/l or more (140 mg/dl in America) if you have fasted overnight, or if the glucose is 11.1 or more (200 mg/dl) if you have eaten, then you have diabetes.

If you have no symptoms of diabetes, two blood samples must show a glucose concentration above these levels before the diagnosis of diabetes can be confirmed.

If your fasting blood glucose is below 6.7 mmol/l (120 mg/dl) or a sample after food is below 7.8 mmol/l (140 mg/dl) you do not have diabetes. There is a grey area in between these figures and those which define diabetes. People whose blood glucose levels fall within this grey area are said to have impaired glucose tolerance. You may return to normal, stay as you are or progress to definite frank diabetes.

The lower limit of normal
This causes confusion. The majority of doctors agree that a blood glucose concentration below 2.2 mmol/1 (40 mg/dl) is definitely abnormally low (i.e. hypoglycaemic) and needs urgent treatment to return it to normal. Each hospital laboratory will produce a normal range for blood glucose based on the thousands of samples it receives – the lower end of this range is usually about 3.5 mmol/1 (63 mg/dl). For practical purposes I suggest that people with diabetes on glucose-lowering treatment regard 4 mmol/l (72 mg/dl) as their lower limit of normal. As your blood glucose falls below this you are more and more likely to feel symptoms of an unduly low blood glucose – hypoglycaemia – and need to eat glucose to correct this.

What should the blood glucose level be?
What should the blood glucose level be in someone who has been diagnosed as diabetic and is being treated? Normal. Nowadays, one of the most important aims in the treatment of diabetes is to return the blood glucose level to normal and keep it there. This is the ideal, and everyone realizes that there are many occasions when a treated diabetic's blood glucose is above normal. Nevertheless, the blood glucose level should be between 3.5 and 7.8 mmol/l (63–140 mg/dl), 4 and 8 for simplicity, and action should be taken if it is always outside this range. It is important not to strive so hard to achieve a normal blood glucose level that your diabetes is overtreated and the level falls too low. This is especially important when you measure your glucose level

before you break your fast after a night's sleep. Attempts by insulin-treated diabetics to keep this at 4 mmol/l (72 mg/dl) may lead to night-time hypoglycaemia; therefore 5 or 6 mmol/l (90 or 108 mg/dl) is safer.

How do I find out what my blood glucose is?

Over the past ten years or so, several companies have developed blood glucose measuring systems. They all rely on a drop of blood from a finger or ear lobe. There are two main methods. In the older, most widely used strip systems, the drop of blood is placed on a pad containing a chemical, glucose oxidase, and dyes. As the glucose in the blood reacts with the glucose oxidase the pigment in the dyes is released causing a colour change on the pad. This colour change can then be read by eye or by placing the strip into a reflectance meter which uses light reflected off the colour to produce a number – the blood glucose concentration. In order to read the colour the blood must be washed (Dextrostix – now rarely used), wiped (BM strips or Chemstrips bG) or blotted (Glucostix) away so that the colour is revealed. The timing is critical – if the blood is left on the pad for too short or too long a time the reading will be inaccurate. Also, if the blood is not removed properly, residual blood may confuse the reading, or the pad may be damaged. If used properly these techniques are very accurate. If you are colour blind, you must use a meter. People with diabetic eye damage may have poor colour vision and should also use a meter. Commonly used meters are Reflolux II and Glucometer II. Hypoguard is another system. All these methods take at least one minute and usually two.

The other system uses a biosensor. The test strip with its test pad is first inserted into the sensor – the smallest are pen-sized or credit card sized. The drop of blood is placed on the pad which is divided into an active pad coated with glucose oxidase and a reference pad. As the glucose in the blood reacts with the glucose oxidase in the active pad, tiny electrical differences occur between this and the reference pad. These are conducted into the biosensor and converted to a number – the blood glucose concentration. This takes 30 seconds. The most commonly used biosensor is Exactech. This system is as accurate as the laboratory, provided the user follows the instructions exactly. A disadvantage is that you cannot check a colour change by eye to make sure that the reading is about right. Advantages are that the blood does not need to be removed and it is quicker.

At present, in the UK, all blood testing strips are available on prescription from general practitioners but meters must be bought. It is wise to look at several systems before paying £40 or more for a meter or biosensor. Consider ease of operation for you, portability, robustness, battery needs, the availability of help from the company and local support. Never buy the first meter you see – for example at a demonstration at a local diabetes group meeting. Never let someone else choose for you.

How should I prick my finger?

Many people are not very enthusiastic about pricking their fingers. There are devices to make it easier and less painful. Autolet II, Monojector and Softouch are automatic finger prickers with a spring to do the pricking (also Lancet in the United States), and they are designed to produce the smallest hole needed to obtain an adequate drop of blood. Some people simply use a little lancet on its own (for example, Monolets, Glucolet II, Unilets) or a fine needle. You can prick the pulp of the finger or the sides of the fleshy part at the base of the nails. Some people prick their ear lobe. Before pricking, wash your hands with soap and warm water, rinse them well and dry them on a clean towel. If they are dirty use an antiseptic swab but make sure that you wipe off all traces of antiseptic with clean absorbent cotton, or cotton wool, or gauze because antiseptic may interfere with the chemical reaction on the testing strip. It is easier to get blood out of a warm finger. A cold room or outside temperature may also cause low glucose results.

Doing a blood glucose test

When doing a blood glucose test, set out what you need before pricking your finger (it saves getting blood everywhere while searching for things). You need:

1. A clean, warm finger or ear lobe
2. a. Glucose testing strips ± your meter
or b. Your Biosensor + strips
3. A lancet or needle and automatic pricker if used
4. Clean cotton wool
5. A watch with a second hand or timer if necessary
6. A water bottle if using Dextrostix
7. Three minutes peace on your own
8. A good light for checking the result.

The blood glucose concentration is in mmol/l in Europe, or in mg/dl in North America; 1 mmol/1 = 18 mg/dl.

Problems with blood glucose testing

Getting blood If you have problems obtaining blood, a quick test can become a prolonged misery. Some people have thicker skin than others – most finger-pricking systems have several different platforms allowing different depths of penetration of the lancet. Some trial and error will help you to find the right depth. If your fingers are cold you will have

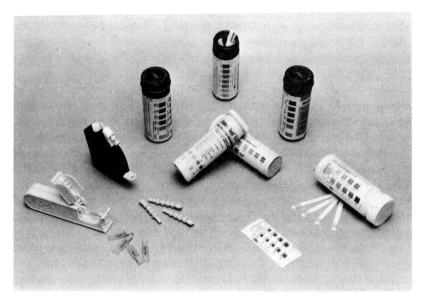

Blood and urine testing: two types of finger pricking devices, urine, glucose and ketone testing strips, blood glucose testing strips and colour matching chart.

trouble obtaining blood. Squeezing the finger tip hard makes it sore and dilutes the blood with serum, giving an unduly low reading. So warm your hands before testing. Milk the blood up from the base of your finger. Another trick to increase blood flow is to shake your hand vigorously with the fingers downwards by your side. See your fingertips go pink. (This is rather like shaking the sauce bottle to get the last drops out!) People with thin skin or who bruise easily need less needle penetration so use a thicker platform. Your fingers should not become sore. If they are ask your diabetic specialist nurse for help.

Inaccurate results   If you do not put the right amount of blood on the test strip you will not obtain an accurate answer. Smearing or dabbing invalidates the result as does drowning the pad in a giant drop. If you mistime the reaction the result will be meaningless – this includes failing to look at your watch or not pressing the button on the meter or biosensor immediately. Failure to press the biosensor button as soon as the blood touches the pad will lead to unduly low readings. Do not tilt the strip or biosensor while the blood drop is on the strip. Cold, heat, wind or rain can all make a nonsense of the result by affecting the glucose oxidase (heat, cold) or by drying out (heat, wind) or diluting the blood drop (rain).

John is 15. He has had diabetes since infancy. He always produces a neat diabetic diary. But his clinic glucose concentrations are always higher than his home tests. One day, away from the hospital, I saw him test his glucose. He pricked his finger, smeared some blood onto the test strip, counted up to sixty out loud, wiped the blood off on his trousers, counted up to sixty (faster this time) and glanced at the strip – "9," he said, casually.

Check points
Are your strips in date? Are they the right ones for your meter? Have you calibrated your meter/biosensor for this particular batch of strips? Is your meter working properly? Have you followed up any error messages? Does it need a new battery?

Have you kept your strips dry and not too cold or too hot? (If you have left the top off the bottle, throw the strips away and start a new pot.) And make sure you put the top on firmly as soon as you have taken a strip out.

Is your equipment clean? Clean meters according to instructions, especially the window through which the strip is read. Biosensors need little cleaning and nothing but the test strip should be placed in the entry port. Is your finger-pricker clean? Change the lancet and platform every time if you wish, although most people reuse platforms if they are the only user. If you are caring for someone else, Glucolet II is a lancet designed to avoid needle-stick injury. Always change lancets and platforms every time if several people are using the same finger-pricker. This avoids transmission of blood-bourne diseases.

The future
Glucose sensors which can be implanted have been available for some time but are still in the experimental stage and tend to be too fragile for everyday use.

There are several meters on the market which have a memory and will hold a variable number of previous blood glucose results. It is likely that this type of meter will be used increasingly. Some meters download this information into a computer held at home or at the diabetes centre. This allows calculation of average blood glucose levels for different times of day, for example.

Glycosylated haemoglobin
A single blood glucose measurement tells you what your glucose level is at that moment. It does not tell you what your glucose level was ten minutes ago or what it was earlier the same day. If you test several times a day and record all your results you can build up a picture of what is happening to your blood glucose level over weeks or months. If you wish, you can calculate your average blood glucose level at a given time of day or throughout a given period, as in the computer system I have just mentioned. Alternatively, hospital clinics are now using a single blood test which can give an indi-

cation of your average blood glucose level over a period of several weeks before the blood was taken. This is the glycosylated haemoglobin or haemoglobin A_{1c} test.

Haemoglobin carries oxygen in the blood stream, inside the red blood cells, and is responsible for their red colour. Each person has several types of haemoglobin including one called haemoglobin A_{1c}. During the 120 days in the life of a red blood cell the haemoglobin A_{1c} (like many other body proteins) is exposed to the prevailing blood glucose levels. Glucose is 'attached' to the haemoglobin A_{1c} to form glycosylated haemoglobin. The percentage of glycosylated haemoglobin depends on how high the blood glucose level has been during the life of the red cells. Different hospital laboratories have different ways of measuring glycosylated haemoglobin, and thus different normal ranges, but as a rough guide, your glycosylated haemoglobin should be below about 8 per cent.

The test is useful as a check on whether finger prick blood tests are giving a representative picture of what is happening to the blood glucose level. It is especially useful for diabetics who rarely or never test their blood glucose level. For example, Mark, who is thirty-nine, works in a horse racing stable and finds that his hands are too dirty to allow finger prick tests. When he went to his clinic, his blood glucose level (from a vein) was 7 mmol/l (126 mg/dl) which looked very good. Then we saw that his glycosylated haemoglobin level was 18 per cent, indicating that he had had very high blood glucose levels over the preceding few weeks. His glucose level was 7 mmol/l that day because he had missed his lunch rushing to get to the clinic. One of the difficulties in interpreting the glycosylated haemoglobin result is that a normal level may represent relatively high blood glucose concentrations alternating with hypoglycaemia. Also, if you are anaemic or have any condition in which the life of the red blood cells is shortened, the result of the test is difficult to interpret. Nevertheless, it is a helpful test and some clinics now use it instead of blood glucose estimations.

Urine glucose tests

What about urine tests? These tests have been the mainstay of self-monitoring for many years. The kidneys help to maintain the normal blood glucose concentration by saving glucose from being excreted. However, the kidneys do not conserve glucose indefinitely and when the blood glucose level rises above the kidney, or renal, threshold (which is slightly different in each person) glucose starts to appear in the urine. This threshold lies at about 10 mmol/l (180 mg/dl) but may occasionally be very different from this. Someone with a very high renal threshold (for example, 15 mmol/l or 270 mg/dl) would have negative urine tests until his blood glucose level rose above 15 mmol/l (270 mg/dl). Someone with a low renal threshold (for example, 4 mmol/l or 72 mg/dl) would sometimes show glucose in the urine

19

URINE

Diet:

MONTH SEPT		~~INSULIN~~ TABLETS		1st Before B/fast	2nd Before B/fast	Before Midday Meal	Before Evening Meal	Before Bed
Day	Date	A.M.	P.M.					
SUN	1	07.30	12.00			0%		
MON	2	08.00	12.30	0%				
TUES	3	07.30	12.30					0%
WED	4	08.00	12.00				0%	
THURS	5	07.30	12.30	0%				
FRI	6	07.15	12.30			0%		
SAT	7	07.30	12.00					0%
SUN	8	08.00	13.00	0%				
MON	9	07.30	12.00				0%	
TUES	10	07.30	12.30			0%		
WED	11	07.30	12.30					0%
THURS	12	08.00	13.00	0%				
FRI	13	07.30	12.00				0%	
SAT	14	07.30	12.30			0%		
SUN	15	08.00	12.30					0%
MON	16	07.30	12.00	0%				
TUES	17	08.00	12.30			0%		
WED	18	07.45	13.00				0%	
THURS	19	08.00	12.30	0%				
FRI	20	07.30	12.30					0%
SAT	21	07.30	12.00			0%		
SUN	22	08.30	13.00				0%	
MON	23	07.30	12.00	0%				
TUES	24	07.00	12.30					0%
WED	25	07.30	12.00			0%		
THURS	26	07.00	12.30				0%	
FRI	27	07.30	12.00	0%				
SAT	28	07.00	12.30			0%		
SUN	29	08.00	13.00					0%
MON	30	07.30	12.30	0%				
	31							
SUMMARY		O		9		8	6	7
Urine Test Results		Trace or ½%		NIL		NIL	NIL	NIL
		1% or 2%						
		3% or 5%						

A urine testing card kept by someone at our clinic who is taking oral hypoglycaemic medication.

even if he were not diabetic. The higher the blood glucose level rises above the renal threshold, the more glucose appears in the urine. High urine glucose concentrations draw water out of the body while the urine is being made, fluid is then lost and you become thirsty. This urine gradually collects in the bladder until it is emptied. The glucose concentration in a urine sample, therefore, represents how much above the renal threshold the blood glucose was during the time it took for the urine to collect in the bladder. Urine tests are therefore:

1. Not as accurate as blood glucose tests because they depend on each person's renal threshold
2. An average, depending on how long the urine has been collecting in the bladder.

Even so, urine tests can be a useful indicator of general glucose control, especially if you know your approximate renal threshold. (You can work this out yourself by comparing blood and urine tests over the same time period.) Many diabetics use both blood and urine tests to monitor their glucose control. For example, if you test the first urine that you pass in the morning, that is, the urine that has been accumulating in your bladder while

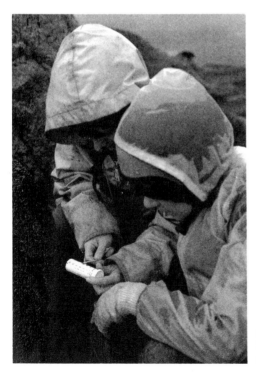

Measuring blood glucose during a mountain expedition; this is simple to do and guards against hypoglycaemia.

21

you are asleep at night, and it shows glucose, you know that for part of the night your blood glucose has been above the renal threshold even if your pre-breakfast glucose is normal. If you find that your fingers are getting sore from finger prick tests, try doing some urine tests instead (but check on your finger prick technique as well; perhaps you are going too deep).

Urine can be tested using strips such as Clinistix, Diastix, Tes-tape and Diabur 5000; in the United States, also Betascan Reagent Strips, Kyodex and Chemstrip uG. Either hold the strip briefly in the urine stream and read after the correct time or you can save urine samples during the day to test at home. As with the blood glucose monitoring strips, it is important that you follow the manufacturer's instructions carefully.

When to do blood or urine tests

You should test your blood or urine whenever you are worried about your diabetes. Do not sit there worrying. Find out what is happening to your blood glucose so that you can do something about it. Experiment by testing after an unusual day, a different meal, a family upset, or a new hobby. See how your moods, your work, your meals and your activities affect your

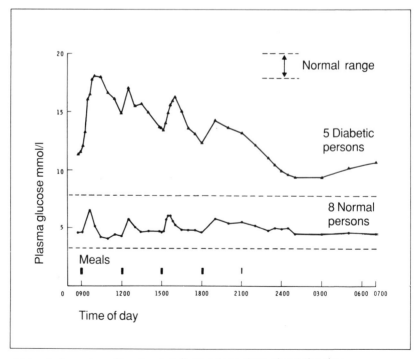

A blood glucose profile showing fluctuations throughout the day.

diabetes. Write the results of your tests down so that you can refer back to them. Many manufacturers provide free diaries in which to do this. When we study diabetics in research projects we may make a twenty-four hour glucose profile. This means that we take a tiny sample of blood every hour from a little plastic tube in a vein and plot the blood glucose level on a graph. A glucose profile is shown in the diagram. Notice the peaks after every meal and the low levels at night. Blood testing every hour is not necessary in day-to-day life and would give you very sore fingers! Most people test the glucose in their blood or urine before each main meal – before breakfast, before lunch, before the evening meal – and also before going to bed. If you test after meals you will have higher results but these should still, ideally, be below 8 mmol/l or 140 mg/dl. Some people test only once a day, but at a different time each day – before breakfast on Monday, before lunch on Tuesday, before the evening meal on Wednesday and so on. It is important to build up a picture of what is happening throughout the day. Discuss the timing of your tests with your doctor.

I thought the idea was to make life easier! It is. You will soon become skilled at testing your blood or urine and it will only take a few minutes. The time spent and the momentary discomfort of finger pricks is well repaid by the peace of mind you gain from knowing what is going on. Why keep yourself in the dark?

Finding out what is happening
- The first step in taking command of your diabetes is to learn how to measure your blood glucose level and to continue to keep a close eye on it.
- The most direct way of doing this is to do finger prick blood glucose tests.
- Urine tests can also be helpful, provided you understand their limitations.
- When you have found out what is happening to your blood glucose level you can use the knowledge to get the very best out of your treatment and to adjust it to suit what you want to do each day.

2 Taking command of your diabetes
Getting the best out of your treatment

Diet

Nowadays, we all know that a diabetic diet, in common with any diet, should have a high fibre content and not include too many saturated fats. It should also contain the correct number of calories to maintain your body weight at the acceptable average for your height, sex and age, or to achieve this level if you are overweight.

The diabetic diet is fundamental to the treatment of diabetes and should be one of the first lessons learned by all new diabetics, whether it is their only treatment or whether they also need oral hypoglycaemic pills or insulin injections. However carefully you manipulate your insulin or oral hypoglycaemic treatment, lack of attention to diet can lead to poor glucose balance both immediately and in the long term.

If you have non-insulin-dependent diabetes it is likely that you are overweight. This makes your body resistant to the action of insulin. The most important part of your treatment is to return to the ideal body weight for your height and stay there, by eating healthy high fibre foods and avoiding sugary foods and excessive amounts of saturated fats.

Nowadays, we all know that a diabetic diet, in common with the diet advised for the whole country, should contain lots of starchy carbohydrate with plenty of fibre, very little saturated fat or sugar and some protein. You should eat the amount needed to keep your weight within the acceptable range for your height. This weight should give you a body mass index of about 22. You can calculate this from your weight in kilogrammes and your height in metres. (1 kg = 2.2 lbs. 1 inch = 2.54 cm.) The body mass index (usually abbreviated to BMI) is your weight divided by your height squared. Thus John who weighs 15 stone (95.5 kg) and is 6 foot (1.83 m) tall has a BMI of 95.5/1.83×1.83 = 28.5. He should weigh 73.7 kg.

At least 55 per cent of the total calories should be starchy carbohydrates or pulses, with over 30g fibre a day, fat should account for less than 35 per cent of the total calories (10 per cent saturated, 20 per cent polyunsaturated or monounsaturated), and between 10–15 per cent protein. Sugar should be less than 4 teaspoons of sucrose or the equivalent, added salt less than 3g daily.

Many of you will have been taught to weigh your food and to count exchanges of carbohydrate, and even of fat or protein. If you feel comfortable with this then continue, but nowadays dietitians are moving away from such rigid dietary control. I once met someone who dipped a urine testing strip into everything she drank to see if it was too sugary. She felt she needed an extremely strict diet to manage her diabetes and became very distressed when she was away from home and unable to calculate her exchanges exactly. She had become a prisoner of her diabetic diet.

The problem is that our bodies are not machines. A car owner can calculate the number of miles his car goes per gallon and knows how much the fuel tank holds – so he knows how much fuel he needs and how often. But there are so many variables in the working of the human body that a simplistic view of food as a fuel may lead to a false sense of security.

For example, if John needs 50 grammes of carbohydrate to work all afternoon, he could eat his 50 g of carbohydrate in various ways – 20 g as new potatoes, 20 g as bread and 10 g as an apple. But if he eats the potato as crisps and the apple as apple juice, the same 50 g of carbohydrate will produce a different rise in his blood glucose after the meal because these foods will be digested differently. It is possible to calculate the amount each carbohydrate containing food will elevate the blood glucose concentration as compared with an equivalent amount of carbohydrate as glucose itself. This produces the glycaemic index. For example, the glycaemic index of new potatoes is 70 but the glycaemic index of potato crisps is 51.

What are the practical implications? If there is such a variable blood glucose response to carbohydrate foods there seems little point in weighing out precise carbohydrate portions for every meal. However, for people taking insulin, it is helpful to have some idea of how much carbohydrate a meal contains as this is one factor which determines how much insulin you inject. It is also helpful for all of us to know approximately what is on our plates in terms of total energy (calories), carbohydrate, fat and protein. Start looking at the back of food packets and the labels on tins – most now provide this information. One piece of useful information is that 1 g of fat provides twice the number of calories (9 cals/g) as 1 g of carbohydrate (3.8 cals/g) or 1 g of protein (4.0 cals/g). Most foods contain water which adds to the weight but not the energy content.

John has a plateful of food containing about 500 calories. Of this 55 per cent (275 cals) should be starchy carbohydrate, 30 per cent (150 cals) should be fat and 15 per cent (75 cals) should be protein. John could eat this as 75 g carbohydrate, 17 g fat and 16 g protein. This is approximately equivalent to 290 g boiled potato (it contains a lot of water) with 100 g lean ham (it contains some water). Lettuce, tomatoes and onion rings, all of which can be regarded as calorie-free could be added, with 20 g salad cream and two apples for dessert.

There is absolutely no need to do such complex dietary calculations yourself – as discussed above this is not appropriate – but this example shows you how tiny your helpings of fatty foods should be in comparison with carbohydrate foods. Essentially your plate should contain four helpings (by weight) of dry carbohydrate food, one helping of fat and one helping of protein.

If your foods have water in them (like vegetables or meat) you can eat more of them than of drier foods. Because protein foods often contain fat you will find there is very little of your fat allowance left over for dressings or spreading on your bread. Some carbohydrate foods also contain fat (potato crisps). This can make them very high in calories (potato crisps contain 559 cals per 100 g, boiled old potatoes 80 cals per 100 g) but may also use up most of your fat allowance (100 g crisps contain 37 g fat).

Special diabetic foods have no place in your diet. They contain fructose or sorbitol and neither has been shown to be of definite benefit in the management of diabetes. You are better eating small amounts of natural foods as part of your diet.

Other books in this series give detailed advice about your diet: *The Diabetics' Diet Book* by Jim Mann and the Oxford Dietetic Group; *The Diabetics' Cookbook* by Roberta Longstaff and Jim Mann; *The High Fibre Cookbook* by Pamela Westland; and *Diabetes: A New Guide* by Rowan Hillson. Excellent information is also available from the American, British and Australian Diabetic Associations and their journals will help to keep you up to date with new dietary ideas.

Insulin

There is now a huge range of insulins for you and your doctor to choose from. Each doctor knows a few insulins well and tends to use them, but

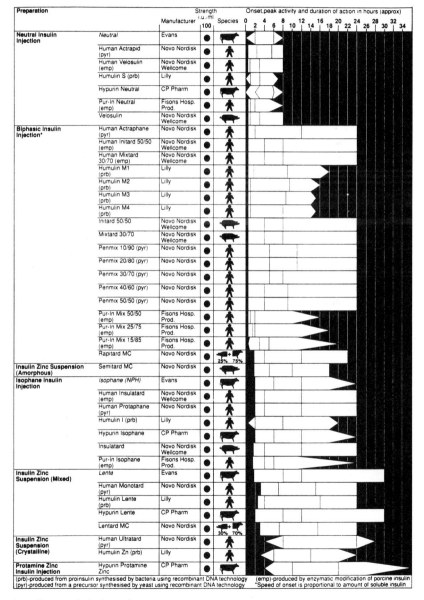

Preparation		Manufacturer	Strength i.u./ml 100	Species	Onset, peak activity and duration of action in hours (approx)
Neutral insulin Injection	Neutral	Evans	●	🐷	
	Human Actrapid (pyr)	Novo Nordisk	●	🚶	
	Human Velosulin (emp)	Novo Nordisk Wellcome	●	🚶	
	Humulin S (prb)	Lilly	●	🚶	
	Hypurin Neutral	CP Pharm	●	🐄	
	Pur-In Neutral (emp)	Fisons Hosp. Prod.	●	🚶	
	Velosulin	Novo Nordisk Wellcome	●	🐷	
Biphasic Insulin Injection*	Human Actraphane (pyr)	Novo Nordisk	●	🚶	
	Human Initard 50/50 (emp)	Novo Nordisk Wellcome	●	🚶	
	Human Mixtard 30/70 (emp)	Novo Nordisk Wellcome	●	🚶	
	Humulin M1 (prb)	Lilly	●	🚶	
	Humulin M2 (prb)	Lilly	●	🚶	
	Humulin M3 (prb)	Lilly	●	🚶	
	Humulin M4 (prb)	Lilly	●	🚶	
	Initard 50/50	Novo Nordisk Wellcome	●	🐷	
	Mixtard 30/70	Novo Nordisk Wellcome	●	🐷	
	Penmix 10/90 (pyr)	Novo Nordisk	●	🚶	
	Penmix 20/80 (pyr)	Novo Nordisk	●	🚶	
	Penmix 30/70 (pyr)	Novo Nordisk	●	🚶	
	Penmix 40/60 (pyr)	Novo Nordisk	●	🚶	
	Penmix 50/50 (pyr)	Novo Nordisk	●	🚶	
	Pur-In Mix 50/50 (emp)	Fisons Hosp. Prod.	●	🚶	
	Pur-In Mix 25/75 (emp)	Fisons Hosp. Prod.	●	🚶	
	Pur-In Mix 15/85 (emp)	Fisons Hosp. Prod.	●	🚶	
	Rapitard MC	Novo Nordisk	●	🐷+🐄 25% 75%	
Insulin Zinc Suspension (Amorphous)	Semitard MC	Novo Nordisk	●	🐷	
Isophane insulin Injection	Isophane (NPH)	Evans	●	🐷	
	Human Insulatard (emp)	Novo Nordisk Wellcome	●	🚶	
	Human Protaphane (pyr)	Novo Nordisk	●	🚶	
	Humulin I (prb)	Lilly	●	🚶	
	Hypurin Isophane	CP Pharm	●	🐄	
	Insulatard	Novo Nordisk Wellcome	●	🐷	
	Pur-In Isophane (emp)	Fisons Hosp. Prod.	●	🚶	
Insulin Zinc Suspension (Mixed)	Lente	Evans	●	🐷	
	Human Monotard (pyr)	Novo Nordisk	●	🚶	
	Humulin Lente (prb)	Lilly	●	🚶	
	Hypurin Lente	CP Pharm	●	🐄	
	Lentard MC	Novo Nordisk	●	🐷+🐄 30% 70%	
Insulin Zinc Suspension (Crystalline)	Human Ultratard (pyr)	Novo Nordisk	●	🚶	
	Humulin Zn (prb)	Lilly	●	🚶	
Protamine Zinc Insulin Injection	Hypurin Protamine Zinc	CP Pharm	●	🐄	

(prb)-produced from proinsulin synthesised by bacteria using recombinant DNA technology
(pyr)-produced from a precursor synthesised by yeast using recombinant DNA technology
(emp)-produced by enzymatic modification of porcine insulin
*Speed of onset is proportional to amount of soluble insulin

Insulins and their action

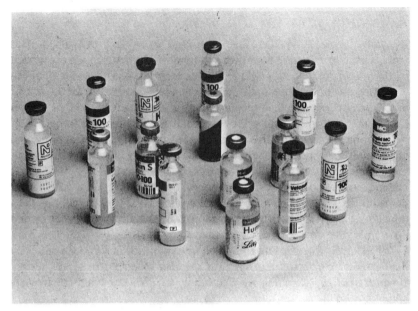

Different types of insulin.

it is important to remember that you do not have to stay on your current insulin regimen if you do not feel that it is suiting you. You need to know as much about your insulin as possible – its name, species, who makes it, how soon it starts to act after an injection, how long its best effect lasts and when its action is finished. Learn what these factors are thought to be by the manufacturers and then find out what happens in your case.

80 per cent of people who take insulin are now using human insulin. Most of this is made by bacteria or yeasts genetically programmed to produce human insulin, but some is made by modification of pork insulin. It is extremely pure and is the same as the insulin non-diabetics make in their bodies. The older beef and pork insulins are still available and pork insulin is highly purified. There has always been concern that animal insulins are more likely to cause antibodies to form in the body. It has been suggested that antibodies may be involved in the development of some tissue damage and that they could, in theory, harm the foetus in utero. Such concerns have not, however, been confirmed in large scientific studies. Antibodies can form to human insulin but this is probably less likely than with insulin from a "foreign" species.

There has been recent concern that people taking human insulin are more likely to experience hypoglycaemia, and that their hypoglycaemic warning symptoms are reduced or altered compared with animal insulin. Human insulin is absorbed more rapidly from the injection site than animal insulin and many people find that they can inject it just before their meal rather than waiting 20 minutes before eating. While there do seem to be some differences in the symptoms of hypoglycaemia in some people, studies have not shown a consistent difference between human and animal insulins. The matter is still under scientific review. If you are worried about your insulin, discuss it with your diabetes doctor straightaway. Your problem may have a simple solution unrelated to your insulin, but if you are still unhappy about being on human insulin then ask to change. It would seem sensible to keep a careful diabetes record before and after such a change so that you can see for yourself whether there has, in fact, been any improvement. (There was a very careful study of people who claimed that their warning symptoms of hypoglycaemia had vanished on human insulin and reappeared on animal insulin. It showed that there was no difference between their symptoms, hormone reponses, or other body responses when made hypoglycaemic on animal and human insulins, on separate occasions under laboratory conditions. The subjects could not tell which insulin was which.) Both human and animal insulins lower the blood glucose effectively and the important issue is whether you feel confident about your insulin treatment.

It certainly seems logical to use human insulin injections to replace missing insulin in humans who cannot make it, rather than injecting foreign insulin from another species. The real problem is that the body "expects" its insulin to arrive in exactly appropriate amounts for the current blood glucose concentration. It "expects" this insulin to be released exactly when needed from the pancreas deep in the abdomen, not gradually trickling into the peripheral circulation from a leg or an arm. It also "expects" insulin release to be reduced as the blood glucose levels fall. But once insulin has been injected into the subcutaneous tissue it will be released into the circulation regardless of blood glucose concentrations. For me, the wonder of insulin treatment is that we can control the blood glucose as well as we can, given the difference between the sophistication of nature and the simplicity of current insulin treatment methods.

Problems with insulin

In theory you inject a known amount of insulin into your leg, it is absorbed in a standard time and reduces the blood glucose by a predictable amount over a given time. Wrong. Your body is not a machine. Firstly, many people (including doctors and nurses) make errors in drawing up their insulin so that 36 units may actually be 34 units on Monday, 35 units on Tuesday, 37 units on Wednesday, 36 units on Thursday, and so on. Pre-mixing in the syringe may alter the characteristics of your insulins – if you mix, say, Monotard and Actrapid, and do not give it immediately, much of the Actrapid will be converted into Monotard before injection. Mixtures of isophane insulins and soluble insulins are stable (eg Velosulin and Insulatard). Then you have to inject the insulin into the subcutaneous tissue below the skin. Not into the skin – that hurts and makes a white bump. Not into the muscle – that hurts and your insulin is absorbed much faster than you expect. Occasionally a trickle of insulin may leak out of the injection hole. The blood supply to the injection site varies – more in hot weather or a warm bath, less in cold water or a cold shower, more when you are exercising – especially if you are using the muscles below your injection site. The nicotine in a cigarette has variable effects upon your circulation.

Damian, a twenty-year-old history student, came home from a class, took his insulin and had a quick bath before his evening meal. He was found unconscious in the bath sometime later. He had become hypoglycaemic because the hot bath water warmed his injection site and the insulin was rapidly absorbed at a time when he was due for a meal.

The insulin also has to break down ready for use. Soluble, regular, clear insulin does not need to do this, but other, cloudy insulins have been treated to slow down their absorption from the injection site. Their crystalline structure may be different or they may have zinc or protamine added. Studies have shown that the amount of isophane insulin left at the injection site 24 hours after a single injection varies from none to 50 per cent of the original dose. There is less variability in the absorption of clear, soluble insulins than of modified insulins. This observation partly explains why some people taking Monotard insulin need to inject it twice a day and others have nocturnal hypoglycaemia following a once-daily pre-breakfast injection. Unfortunately, the absorption is not always consistent for one person and may vary from day to day.

Obviously insulin is not the only factor influencing the blood glucose – food, exercise, your weight, general fitness, hormone state, other medication, illness, stress and so on can also affect glucose concentrations.

Which insulin regimen might suit you?

Fixed proportion mixtures
These are mixtures of clear, soluble, fast-acting insulin and cloudy, isophane, medium-acting insulin made by the manufacturer. Mixtures

(fast:medium) include 10:90, 20:80, 30:70, 40:60, 50:50. The advantages are that you do not need to mix them so it is quicker for you, there is less possibility of error in making up the mixture, they are more convenient. There are sufficient variations to allow a different insulin morning and evening and adjustments to your life-style. The disadvantage is that you have no control over the proportions in the mixture on any one occasion. Thus you may be planning a football game one afternoon and would prefer to reduce the morning dose of isophane insulin. But you have to reduce the whole mixture and may find yourself sugary before lunch because you also reduced the dose of fast-acting insulin. Fixed proportion mixtures have grown in popularity and in practice many people find them satisfactory for most of the time. I would always start a person with new diabetes on a fixed proportion mixture to make it easier for them at first.

Fast and medium separately twice a day
This usually means soluble insulin (eg Actrapid, Humulin S or Velosulin) and an isophane insulin (eg Humulin I, Insulatard, Protaphane), but some people may inject a longer-acting insulin such as Monotard twice a day. The advantage of this regimen is that you have four insulin peaks to adjust – morning fast insulin working until lunch-time, morning medium insulin working during the afternoon, evening fast insulin working until bed-time, evening medium insulin working through the night to breakfast-time. This makes it very flexible. The disadvantage is that you have to draw up a precise mixture and there is more possibility of error than with a fixed proportion mixture.

Fast before meals and medium or long before bed
This is the most flexible regimen of all. It is usually used with an insulin pen but people who prefer needles and syringes can use it too. Fast-acting insulin is given before each meal in a dose calculated on the prevailing blood glucose, the amount and timing of the meal and any planned exercise. Medium (eg isophane) or very long-acting insulin (eg Ultratard) is given before bed to cover the night. Some people can miss meals or vary the times at which they eat, others find that they still need to eat regularly. This regimen can improve blood glucose control, but only if you pay attention to your blood glucose results measured before each meal and before bed.

Once daily insulin
It is rarely possible to control a truly insulin-dependent diabetic's blood glucose on once daily insulin. It may stabilise glucose control in someone with type II (maturity onset) diabetes who is still making a little insulin, but not enough for his oral hypoglycaemic pills to work

fully. Sadly, there are still people on once-daily insulin, often those who have diabetes for many years, who refuse to try twice daily insulin injections despite obviously poor glucose balance. They usually have diabetic tissue damage. In someone who is unable to give his or her own insulin injections and who is reliant on the district nurse or a carer who comes once a day, once daily insulin may be the only solution. In this situation one may be aiming for freedom from symptoms of unduly high or unduly low glucose rather than normoglycaemia (a normal blood glucose).

Adjusting your insulin dose

It is your diabetes and you are the person who has to live with it. The sooner you get used to adjusting your own insulin dose the better. I am astounded by the number of diabetics who know that their glucose control is poor but who wait, sometimes for months, until their next appointment for the doctor to tell them to increase their insulin. Many diabetics are afraid that a small change in their insulin dose will cause a catastrophic hypoglycaemic reaction. It is most unusual for this to happen. I usually suggest that anyone who needs to alter the insulin dose starts by adjusting it by one unit at the appropriate time and watches what happens over the next two or three days, making further one unit changes as needed after this. Gradually, most diabetics find that they can make adjustments of two, three or four units at a time if necessary. Discuss how you should set about adjusting your insulin dose with your doctor or diabetic adviser.

I need hardly say that you should reduce your insulin if you are suffering hypoglycaemic episodes and increase it if your blood glucose level is high. If you are taking a combination of insulins you must consider which one is acting at that particular time.

Adjusting your diet

In trying to correct a low or high blood glucose level at a given time of day, it may be simpler, or more appropriate, to adjust your diet rather than your insulin or pills. Perhaps you are using extra energy at that time and need an extra snack. But beware of a common trap – too much insulin makes you hungry or hypoglycaemic, so you eat more and your glucose level goes up, then you take more insulin and get hungry again, then you eat more and get fat and become even more resistant to the action of insulin. Perhaps the timing of your meals or snacks could be modified.

Energetic Ed attends our clinic. He has succeeded in adjusting his diet to suit a varied and very active life.

Ed is twenty-four years old and works as a general builder and decorator. He is a very athletic man; he plays tennis several times a week, plays football most weekends and plays the drums in a rock group. He has been diabetic for four years and has never let his diabetes get in his way. He takes rapid-acting and medium-acting insulin twice daily – sixteen units Velosulin and twenty-eight units Insulatard in the morning and ten units Velosulin with eighteen units Insulatard in the evening.

One Monday morning he was going to demolish a brick wall as part of a renovation scheme on a large project. He knew that this would use more energy than, for example, painting or carpentry. That morning therefore, he reduced his fast-acting Velosulin by four units and not only ate a larger breakfast than usual (double helpings of cereal, and an extra slice of toast) but took an extra snack to eat during the morning. He always plays tennis on Monday nights so his usual food and insulin were already adjusted for that.

The following day Ed's job was to prepare some of the outside woodwork for painting. Because this was less energetic, he had his usual insulin and food that morning. However, at lunchtime he played an unexpected and vigorous game of football with his mates and ate his emergency biscuits from the tin he always keeps in his toolbox. That night his rock group were booked to play at a birthday party. Ed puts everything he's got into the drumming! He reduced his evening Velosulin to eight units and, because it was a late night party, reduced his Insulatard to sixteen units. He ate his usual evening meal but had a snack while he was setting up the amplifiers at the party. He also ate some bread, cheese and fruit at the party. He restricted his beer intake to one pint (unlike the rest of the group) because he had had a bad hypoglycaemic attack two years previously after a similar party when he drank too much and ate too little and his glucose fell during the night. When he finally got home at three in the morning he had a bowl of cereal before he went to bed.

Insulin injection techniques

Disposable syringes and needles
For ease and comfort, disposable plastic syringes with fine-bore disposable needles are best. These are commonly re-used but I have to point out that the manufacturers of disposable syringes and needles describe them as being for single use only and do not recommend re-use. Keep your spare syringes and needles securely in a dry, clean place.

Buttons

Some companies make tiny needles with a small rubber stopper through which you can inject insulin. One of these needles is inserted every one or two days and either taped down or fixed with its own sticky disc and the insulin is injected as needed. A student on one of our outdoor courses had a button that remained in place in her arm while she was canoeing, climbing and scrambling about the ropes course, with no problem at all, despite my secret worries. These buttons are useful for people who need several injections a day and do not like sticking the needle in frequently.

Insulin pens

These are gradually replacing needle and syringe for many people with diabetes. They use a cartridge of insulin instead of an ink cartridge and a double-ended very fine needle instead of a nib. The cartridge is inserted into the barrel of the pen and the needle is screwed onto the pen so that one end pierces the bung of the cartridge. The pen then has to be primed – that is the plunger makes contact with the cartridge's upper bung and all the air (if any) is expelled from the cartridge and needle. The insulin dose is then dialled up and injected (Accupen, BD-

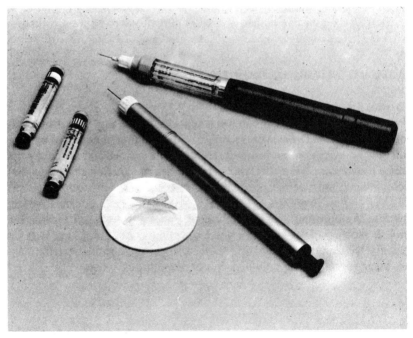

Insulin injection pens, insulin cartridges and a button needle (covered) with an adhesive disc.

Lilly pen, Novopen II, Penmix, Pur-in pen) or the plunger is depressed the appropriate number of times (Novopen I). It is very important that you have a full training session in the use of your pen, and especially that you know how to change cartridges and prime it. Most pens require you to expel air and a tiny squirt of insulin before each use to ensure that it is working. You must keep an eye on the remaining insulin – you may not be able to give your full dose if the cartridge is nearly empty. Find out who your support is if there are problems. This is usually the diabetes specialist nurse but there may also be a company help-line. What would you do if your pen was broken or stolen? Keep a spare pen if you can, if not keep some ordinary insulin and syringes for emergencies. Remember that small or rural pharmacies not be able to supply cartridges easily, and they may be impossible to obtain abroad. At present all pens are manually operated but companies are experimenting on electrically driven pens.

Penject is a device that looks like a large fountain pen. Inside you can fit an ordinary plastic disposable syringe with a needle, replacing the plunger stem of the syringe with the one belonging to the device. A twist of the dial at the top pushes the plunger down to expel two units of U100 insulin. The advantage of this device is that you can fill the syringe with fast-acting insulin and another Penject with slow-acting insulin and carry them in your pocket. At injection time you simply stick the needle under the skin (subcutaneously) as usual and dial in the amount of insulin you need.

Penpump, or in the United States Markwell Pen Pump, is a similar device, which is attached to tubing leading to a fine needle. This is inserted subcutaneously every twenty-four hours, and sometimes at longer intervals, and left there. The device can be hung from a bra strap or put in an inside pocket and the dial can be turned to inject insulin whenever needed. This is really only suitable for fast-acting insulin.

Continuous subcutaneous insulin infusion pumps

The new device that everyone asks about is the continuous subcutaneous insulin infusion (CSII) pump. This is the first step towards the portable artificial pancreas. Put simply, the pancreas needs to be able to do two things as far as the diabetic is concerned. First, to sense the blood glucose level. Second, to increase or decrease insulin output in response to that glucose level. People involved in diabetes research in Japan, and elsewhere, have succeeded in making a fine needle sensor that can be inserted subcutaneously to register the concentration of blood glucose in tiny blood vessels (capillaries). This device can then activate an insulin pump to release the correct amount of insulin. As yet this is not ready for widespread use. There are teething troubles with the glucose sensing part of the artificial pancreas. The insulin infusing part is, though, already on the market.

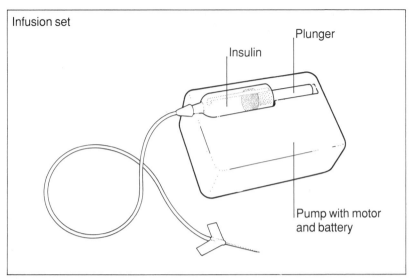

Infusion set

Insulin

Plunger

Pump with motor
and battery

Above, diagram showing how the insulin pump works. *Below*, placing the infusion set in position is a simple operation.

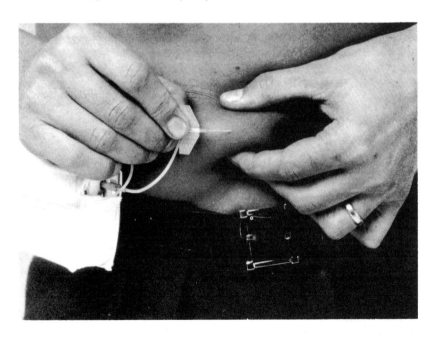

Insulin infusion pumps slowly and continuously push down the plunger of a syringe or vial of insulin at a preset rate. Extra squirts of insulin can be given through a button on the pump, whenever necessary Fast-acting insulin is always used. The pump is set up so that it delivers a background or basal infusion over a twenty-four hour period, then at each meal and sometimes at snack times the wearer presses the button to give the correct amount of insulin to cope with that particular meal. Sally, for example, is on a base rate of twelve units per twenty-four hours (or 0.5 units per hour). She has four units before breakfast, four before lunch and six before her evening meal, which is the largest of the day.

Implantable pumps Heart pacemakers – whose technology is being used to develop CSII pumps – are implanted under the skin. This approach has been tried with a specially adapted CSII pump, which is entirely buried beneath the skin. The pump has a flexible reservoir that can be filled with insulin injected through the skin and the wall of the reservoir. Its batteries keep the small pump going and it can be programmed by external computer, another contribution from pacemaker technology. This device is still at the research stage.

Advantages of CSII The advantages of the pump are that it gives insulin all the time and that it can easily be adjusted to cope with different activities, different meals and early or late meals. Insulin delivery can be as flexible as you want. The insulin release is more like that of the pancreas than the one or two injections of insulin a day. Used properly, it can give normal blood glucose levels throughout the day and night. (So can conventional insulin injections when used carefully.) It has been suggested that CSII may reduce diabetic tissue damage but there is no longterm proof of this.

New models, about the size of two matchboxes side by side, are small enough to hang on a belt or put in a pocket without attracting attention. The most up-to-date models are operated by microcomputer and many variations in insulin dose and timing of administration can be programmed into them. All models have safety features, which is why they cost so much. They can warn of tube kinking or blockage, an empty syringe, and a runaway pump (see below). They can be taken off for an hour or two when you bathe or exercise and the tubing and needle are usually changed every one or two days.

Disadvantages of CSII There are several disadvantages to CSII. The pumps cost a lot of money. The needle is under the skin all the time, always attached to the pump, which in turn is always attached to you. Great care is needed with glucose balance, so frequent blood glucose measurements have to be made. The batteries have to be kept charged because hyperglycaemia, often progressing to ketoacidosis, is rapid if the pump breaks down and stops for more than a few hours; although hypoglycaemia does not seem to be any more common during CSII than with ordinary insulin injections. Pump motors only very occasionally run away and squirt all the insulin in at once because the manufacturers have now taken steps to deal with this problem.

Weigh it up At present the pump is mostly used for diabetics who need especially tight glucose control and cannot achieve this with standard insulin injections. For some diabetics CSII has given them freedom from the tyranny of their diabetes. For others it has given them a lot of trouble and a sore abdomen. Pump therapy should be very carefully discussed with your doctor and, once started, carefully supervised by you and your diabetic adviser, with frequent blood glucose checks. Full time back-up (twenty-four hours, seven days a week) is necessary from a medical team who know how to sort out pump problems. Current forms of CSII are gradually finding their place in treatment and may be the method that suits you. If you are having problems with control or if you think that the pump sounds like a good idea for you, discuss it with your doctor, and weigh up its good and bad points for yourself. If you and your doctor think that the pump may help you, try one first before you buy it. Most companies will lend you a pump for a month to see if it suits you.

Insulin injection sites
All diabetics know that you should inject insulin into the fatty tissue under the skin (subcutaneously) and rotate your injection sites. Antiseptics make the skin hard and the injections sore and so they are best avoided provided your skin is clean. However, people can become so intent on the details of insulin dose adjustment that they forget that one reason why their diabetes is hard to control may be the injection site.

Dents and lumps Nowadays fewer diabetics are taking beef insulin. Most people coming to our clinic take human insulin and the others take highly purified pork insulins. Few use beef insulin. One of the problems with the old beef insulins was fat atrophy (tissue loss) or hypertrophy (tissue gain) at the injection site. These dents and lumps in the thighs or arms can be very unsightly and may also affect the absorption of insulin from that site. Fat atrophy and hypertrophy are considered to be allergic reactions to the insulin and are less common on highly purified human or pork insulins, though they do occur. You can probably lose dents and lumps by changing to human or highly purified pork insulin, if you are not already taking it, and injecting this into the edge of the abnormal area, gradually moving in towards the middle as the problem is resolved. However, it has to be said that this may not cure everyone. The best way to prevent dents and lumps occurring is to rotate your injection sites so that no area is overused.

Ten years ago I met Albert, sixty-three years old, who had been admitted to the hospital because his blood glucose was very poorly controlled. When I examined him I discovered two little black holes, one on the front of each thigh. This was where he had been injecting his insulin for the past five years! Many diabetics have a favourite area for insulin injections, easy to reach and a little numb from years of injections. That is how insulin atrophy and hypertrophy develop.

Red spots and bruises It is not unusual for new diabetics to find little red spots at the site of recent insulin injections. This normally settles down after a few months. But persistent sore red spots or lumps may mean that you are allergic to your current insulin or to the zinc in it. A single very tender lump, which may or may not be red to start with, may be an injection site abscess. This may need lancing and/or antibiotic treatment by your doctor. Bruising at the injection site should not occur very often. If it does, you may be going in too deep. Avoid piercing veins near the surface – you can see them as blue lines.

Oral hypoglycaemic drugs

Pills which reduce the blood glucose level are commonly used in Britain but less frequently in North America, although they are now becoming more widely available there. They are of two main types: sulphonylurea drugs such as chlorpropamide, glibenclamide, gliclazide glipizide, glucuronide; and the biguanides of which the only form in current use is metformin. Sulphonylureas act by increasing both pancreatic insulin production and the use of glucose in tissues. Metformin has no effect on insulin production but reduces glucose absorption from the gut and improves its utilisation at tissue level. Therefore, pills are only useful for people with diabetes who are still producing their own insulin, even though in insufficient quantities. Sometimes a sulphonylurea is combined with metformin. Different sulphonylurea drugs act for different lengths of time, for example, chlorpropamide is very long-acting and taken once a day, whereas glipizide and tolbutamide are short-acting and are taken one to three times a day. Other sulphonylureas are taken once or twice a day. Adjustment of the dose of pills is possible, although to a lesser extent than for insulin injection. While there is no upper limit to the dose of insulin and it can be increased as necessary according to blood glucose measurements, there are maximum safe doses of pills. It is important that you know what these are before considering adjusting your own dose. Each agent will also have its own dose range and practical way of altering the dose (for example, it may be difficult to break some pills in half). It may take several days before you notice any effect from a change in your pill dose (chlorpropamide takes about a week). Ask your doctor about the characteristics of your particular oral hypoglycaemic drug and how you could adjust the dose yourself. It is more common to need an increase in dose than a decrease, but people on oral agents can develop hypoglycaemia and any suspicion of this should lead to an immediate dose reduction and a prompt discussion with your adviser. One in three people taking glibenclamide experience hypoglycaemia.

In order to use your pills effectively consider how they work. The pill has to be swallowed, its covering is digested away and then it dissolves in digestive juices. It is gradually absorbed through the intestinal wall into the blood stream. It then has to travel to where it acts. On the way from the intestine it will pass through the liver and some of it may be removed and broken down at this point. The blood drug levels may not peak for one or two hours (or longer in the case of chlorpropamide) after you have swallowed it. Gradually over the next day or so, the drug will be broken down and cleared from the body. Most sulphonylureas are cleared by the kidney and so levels will build up in the blood stream if your kidneys are not working properly. This increases the risk of hypoglycaemia. Gliquidone and gliclazide are primarily cleared by the liver and these, and the shorter-acting tolbutamide are better for people with kidney disease (although caution is still necessary). Older people are at higher risk of hypoglycaemia and chlorpropamide and glibenclamide are usually avoided in the elderly. Gliclazide, glipizide or tolbutamide may be better.

Because pills have to be absorbed from the gut before they can work, anything that upsets absorption may interfere with their action. This may include a stomach or bowel operation years ago. Diarrhoea and vomiting are obvious problems (see page 52) but taking them after a big meal may delay absorption. Some foods may slow their absorption more than others. Taking them on an empty stomach can irritate the stomach in some people. You must never take them and then not eat. Instructions for taking sulphonylureas vary depending on which book one reads. Most suggest with the meal – I interpret this as swallowing them when you have eaten some, but not all of your food – for example, between the cereal and the toast, or, at dinner time, between the soup and the main course. Wash your pills down with a drink of water or other non-alcoholic beverage.

If your pills are prescribed twice a day, then take them twice a day. With oral hypoglycaemic pills this usually means with breakfast and with your evening meal – but if you are taking tolbutamide or glipizide it may mean with breakfast and lunch – so ask your doctor. It is rare to need more pills with the evening meal than with the morning meal. Too much sulphonylurea at night increases the risk of nocturnal hypoglycaemia. But I do see one man who eats very little in the day and a great deal in the evening who needs 80 mg gliclazide with breakfast and 160 mg gliclazide with his evening meal. This sort of adjustment is only possible in someone who is monitoring their blood glucose carefully. If you take your pills at the wrong time, or take them all at once when you have been advised to divide them you run the considerable risk of hypoglycaemia.

Pill treatment is described in detail in *Diabetes: A new guide* and *Diabetes beyond 40* both by Dr Rowan Hillson.

Getting the best out of your treatment
- Diet is the basis of all treatment for diabetes.
- If you are on additional treatment learn everything you can about it.
- If you are taking insulin:

  1. Learn how fast and for how long each of your insulins acts – both theoretically and in your own case.
  2. Gain confidence in adjusting your own insulin dose.
  3. Consider advances in insulin injection techniques.
  4. Consider whether you have injection site problems.

- If you are taking oral hypoglycaemic pills:

  1. Learn how fast and for how long your pills act.
  2. Learn the maximum safe dose of your pills and consider making adjustments within this maximum.

- Do not be upset if you cannot control your diabetes on pills and diet. The need for insulin treatment is not a disaster and you will learn how to cope with it very quickly.

3 Sorting out problems with glucose balance

Hypoglycaemia

Hypoglycaemia is preventable. Indeed, most attacks severe enough to require medical attention could have been avoided with a little forethought. Most people with diabetes have good warning symptoms that their blood glucose is falling. Learn what yours are as soon as possible. They may be more subtle than you realise. One way of considering the symptoms of hypoglycaemia is to divide them into changes in emotions, changes in thinking, changes in movement, and adrenaline symptoms. You are unlikely to notice changes in conscious level yourself until glucose wakes you up.

Changes in emotion are often inappropriate for the situation. You may be irritable, sad, excited, giggly, withdrawn, angry, frustrated, cheerful or feel you can conquer anything.

Changes in thinking occur before most people realise what is happening. Slowness or difficulty in making decisions is a characteristic feature of a falling glucose. Time seems to slow down. Your ability to calculate, think logically and plan can be impaired. This is why it is so dangerous to drive or operate machinery when you are hypoglycaemic.

Changes in movement may be late symptoms. They include problems with coordinating movement, whether of the throat and mouth to produce coherent speech; coordination of hand movements to draw or do up buttons; or coordination of legs and feet to walk straight, for example. Muscles may become weak and rarely if you have a bad hypoglycaemic episode it can seem as if you have had a stroke. Glucose cures it straightaway. While you might expect lack of glucose to make people slow down, occasionally people seem to have superhuman strength and do things which they would normally find difficult – lifting heavy objects, running up hill, for example.

Adrenaline symptoms are what many people rely on to warn them of hypoglycaemia. Unfortunately these can be late features of a low glucose and it is important to learn *all* your warning symptoms so as to identify the onset of a hypoglycaemic attack as soon as possible. We all know that adrenaline is the fright, flight and fight hormone, hence the pounding rapid heartbeat, the trembling hands and the drenching sweat. Changes in conscious level are uncommon. You may simple feel sleepy, or rarely become unconscious. Although it is rare and the vast majority of people with diabetes treat their minor hypoglycaemic episodes quickly and efficiently with glucose, hypoglycaemic coma is what many non-diabetics associate with diabetes. After all, from the film producer's point of view, it is much more dramatic for the heroine to collapse unconscious in the hero's arms, than for her to say, "I feel a bit hypo", eat some glucose and carry on dancing.

If you have good warning of hypoglycaemia and can learn to recognise your symptoms of a falling glucose, you should have few problems with hypoglycaemia. As the years pass some people on insulin lose their warning symptoms of hypoglycaemia. This happened to Dr Lawrence, the co-founder of the BDA – his junior doctors used to feed him glucose when they noticed that he was hypoglycaemic. Other factors which may reduce your warning are treatment with beta blocker drugs such as propranolol and the level at which your blood glucose concentrations run. If you habitually have a glucose of 10 mmol (180 mg/dl) or more, you are likely to have more intense warning symptoms of hypoglycaemia than someone whose glucose levels are usually between 4 and 8 mmol/l (72–144 mg/dl). This is one reason why people whose blood glucose is persistently high may resist returning it to normal – an understandable reaction. However, the fear of failing to recognise hypoglycaemia must be weighed against the risk of developing the diabetic complications which are linked with a persistently high blood glucose.

Once you have recovered from a hypoglycaemic attack, whether mild or severe, work out why it happened so that you can avoid another one. Did you have too much insulin or too many tablets? Did you eat enough? Did you exercise more than you expected? Were you careless? Seek your diabetes adviser's help if you cannot work out how to prevent another hypoglycaemic attack. If you have been hypoglycaemic on sulphonylurea pills, contact your diabetes adviser that day, as soon as you have eaten.

A rare but distressing problem for a few people with insulin-treated diabetes is that of frequent hypoglycaemia, often without warning. Because hypoglycaemia causes amnesia, you may forget a bad hypoglycaemic attack. But it can worry your family. Listen to their concerns. If you are having frequent hypoglycaemia you must act. First, stop driving and do not do anything which might put you or others in danger. This may mean taking time off work. Next reduce all your insulin by at least one third. You are aiming to have all your blood glucose levels between about 8 and 12 mmol/l (144–216 mg/dl) for a few days or weeks to make certain you cannot have a hypoglycaemic attack. Eat three meals and three snacks each day with a big pre-bedtime snack. Contact your diabetes adviser now to help regain the fine tuning of your glucose balance. This problem can be resolved – it is an emergency. Act now to restore your blood glucose balance and your peace of mind.

Hypoglycaemic attacks are less common among people who take sulphonylurea pills than those treated with insulin. However, they do happen and people taking long-acting pills such as chlorpropamide can, very rarely, have an attack lasting several hours. More often, you simply feel very hungry before the next meal or perhaps a little light-headed. Older people should note that feeling a bit muddled or not quite yourself may be an effect of the hypoglycaemic pills and not of old age! The important thing is to realize that people taking pills to control diabetes can occasionally become hypoglycaemic, so if you feel unwell in any way, consider a low blood glucose level as a possible cause of your feeling.

It goes without saying that anyone with diabetes on insulin or hypoglycaemic pills should carry glucose or some form of carbohydrate all the time. Eat glucose the instant you suspect you are hypoglycaemic. If you are unsure and feel well enough to test, check your blood glucose level. However, remember that the longer you delay treating hypoglycaemia, the harder you may find it to treat. Many people with diabetes have an illogical aversion to food when they are hypoglycaemic and refuse to eat, even though another part of your brain is telling you that you should. This split brain phenomenon is a feature of hypoglycaemia. I was made hypoglycaemic in a research experiment. At the end my colleagues gave me some food. Ugh! Part of my brain told me that the food looked horrible and that I didn't want it and wasn't going to eat it. Another part of my brain told me that I needed food because I was low. A third part said, 'this is interesting, people with diabetes do this when they are hypo, will she overcome the aversion to food or not?' I eventually ate the food with some firm persuasion from my colleagues and my three minds merged to my usual one!

Your family or friends will feel more secure with a supply of glucagon to hand. This hormone reverses the effect of insulin and raises the blood glucose temporarily by releasing glucose from liver stores, awakening you so that you can take food. It can be injected subcutaneously, intramuscularly or intravenously and most people can be taught how to give it. Glucagon keeps for many years, but the expiry date should be checked.

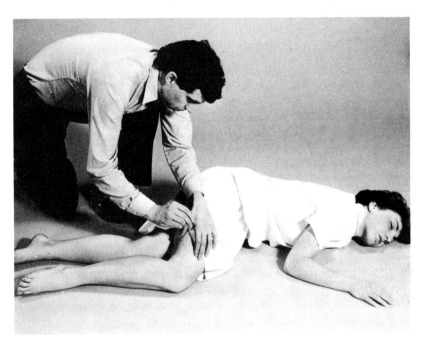

Treating someone unconscious from hypoglycaemia: she is safe lying in the recovery position while you decide calmly what to do. Her companion is about to inject Glucagon into the muscles of her thigh. When she has woken up, give her something to eat.

Someone unconscious from hypoglycaemia should be placed in the recovery position, that is, lying on his or her side with a clear airway. Sometimes, rubbing a glucose tablet or a small quantity of glucose gel inside the cheek and lips will wake someone up from a hypoglycaemic reaction, but do not allow him to choke on it, and be careful to avoid getting bitten.

Severe hyperglycaemia

Theoretically, all blood glucose levels above the normal range represent hyperglycaemia. The occasional value outside this range is no cause for concern. This section is about very high blood glucose levels, persistent values above 13 mmol/l (234 mg/dl) or frequent readings of 22 mmol/l (396 mg/dl) or more. There are many reasons for high blood glucose concentrations, a common one being infection, whether bacterial or viral. At the first signs of illness, start to measure your blood glucose frequently. It may rise even though you are unable to eat. Your insulin requirements may also increase as you become more resistant to the action of insulin while your body fights the infection. It is sensible to plan what you would do if this

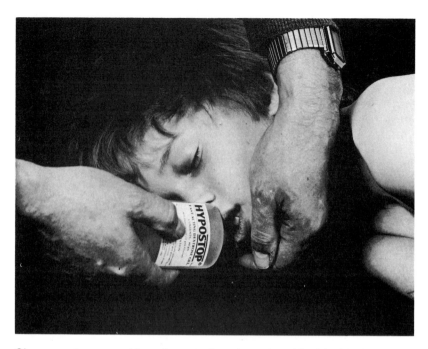

Glucose gel squeezed into the mouth and gently rubbed inside the cheek is another way of helping someone to recover from a hypoglycaemic attack. Be very careful to ensure that she cannot choke.

were to happen and discuss this with your doctor. Write the plan down. When you are feeling ill it is easier to consult the plan than try to remember all the details.

Insulin-treated diabetes

If your glucose level starts to rise, give yourself more insulin. But supposing I take more insulin and then I don't feel like eating? I will make myself hypoglycaemic! How much insulin should I take and when? There are many ways of solving this problem and there is no single correct solution. The only rules are:

1. Never stop your insulin injections
2. Ask for help sooner rather than later.

The simplest and probably the safest way of coping is to continue your long-acting insulin, reducing the dose if necessary, and give extra short-acting insulin in doses of a few units, for example, two to four units, at frequent intervals, perhaps every four hours, according to your blood glucose measurements. Urine tests are not a very good guide at a time like this, when glucose levels may be changing rapidly.

David, who is twenty and has been diabetic since he was four years old, takes Actrapid (short-acting) and Monotard (long-acting) insulin twice a day. He measures his blood glucose level four times daily and usually has values of 4 to 7 mmol/l (72 to 126 mg/dl). He recently had an episode of abdominal cramps, diarrhoea and nausea associated with poor glucose balance. The table shows how he coped with this at home. On Thursday he telephoned me because he still felt ill and his glucose levels were not returning to normal. I saw him that evening and admitted him to the hospital with suspected appendicitis. Fortunately, everything settled down, his glucose control improved and he went home. Throughout his illness his careful management ensured that his blood glucose level never rose above 17 mmol/l (306 mg/dl). When he felt that things were not settling, he sensibly asked for help. I asked him to contact me earlier should this happen again.

When changing your insulin dose or adding extra doses it is important to remember that your clear, fast-acting insulin is the one which will reduce a high glucose over the next few hours. Cloudy insulins have a longer and less predictable onset and duration of action. When adding extra doses of clear, fast-acting insulin, remember to consider whether any other insulin you have injected earlier will be starting to work at that time. Use this information to help calculate the right insulin dose. If you are unsure, contact your diabetic specialist nurse, or doctor for help, there and then.

If your blood glucose is high try to work out why so that you can prevent it from happening again. Apart from the obvious reasons of too little insulin, too much food and too little exercise, consider infection, a reaction to injury, operation or stress, pregnancy, period times, and drugs or medicines. Steroid drugs (e.g. prednisolone) usually increase the blood glucose, thiazides, other diuretics (water pills) and tricyclic antidepressants may do so.

Ketoacidosis
Hyperglycaemia and dehydration   If someone with diabetes is seriously insulin-deficient, various major biochemical changes occur. Without insulin, glucose cannot enter your body cells to be stored or to produce energy. Your body therefore behaves as if you were starving. While a starving man has no glucose available because he has not eaten any, the diabetic has plenty of glucose available but it cannot get into the cells without the help of insulin. The lack of insulin causes the liver to release glucose from its stores,

47

How David coped with his diabetes during his illness

David's usual insulin dose is:
Morning Actrapid (AR) 10 units, Monotard (MT) 18 units;
Evening Actrapid (AR) 4 units, Monotard (MT) 10 units.

Day	Blood glucose level mmol/1	Urine ketones	Insulin
Tuesday			
Before breakfast	4	N/T	AR 10 u
Ate meal			MT 18 u
Before lunch	7	N/T	
Ate meal			
Abdominal cramps + nausea			
Before evening meal	10	+	AR 4 u
Ate glucose only			MT 10u
Before bed	13	+	AR 2 u
Ate small snack			
Vomited during night	10	N/T	—
Wednesday			
Before breakfast	17	++	AR 12 u
Ate small meal			MT 18 u
Abdominal cramps + diarrhoea			
Before lunch	13	++	AR 6 u
Ate lunch then vomited			
Midafternoon	7	+	—
Before evening meal	10	+	AR 4 u
Ate a little			MT 10 u
Before bed	10	+	AR 2 u
Ate snack			
Thursday			
Before breakfast	7	+	AR 10 u
Ate meal			MT 18 u
Before lunch	10	+	—
Severe abdominal cramps	13	+	AR 4 u
Vomiting			
Telephoned for medical help			

N/T = not tested for ketones;
Some snacks omitted to save space.

but of course this cannot be used any better than the glucose derived from the carbohydrates you have eaten. Your blood glucose levels rise, sometimes to 50 mmol/l (900 mg/dl) or more. Glucose starts pouring out into your urine and the thick syrupy fluid draws water out of your body with it. You become more and more dehydrated and however much you drink you cannot keep up with the fluid loss. If you have severe diabetic ketoacidosis you may be short of as much as ten litres (18 pints) of salty water! Potassium starts leaking out of your cells and is passed out in the urine.

Ketones Because your cells are now starving, your body turns to other sources of energy such as proteins and fats. You start to lose weight. Fats are broken down into fatty acids which are, in turn, broken down into ketone bodies. Ketones give the breath a characteristic smell of pear drops and are also passed out in the urine where they can be detected by simple tests (Ketostix, Acetest, Ketur test). As the ketones build up in the blood stream, your blood gradually becomes acid. The build up of acid stimulates the lungs to breathe too hard to blow off acid as carbon dioxide. Gradually your breathing becomes deeper and longer with a sighing quality and a pungent smell of ketones. This deep sighing breathing is called acidotic or Kussmaul breathing and is a classical sign of diabetic ketoacidosis. As the blood becomes increasingly more acid, more biochemical processes fail because they cannot work in an acid environment.

Slow deterioration This takes several hours or days. By now you are feeling very ill. You are vomiting, desperately thirsty, breathing deeply and becoming confused or even semiconscious. You are also very silly to have let your condition get this far without seeking help! Dial for an ambulance and get yourself to a hospital immediately. Surveys in Britain and North America showed that ketoacidosis was the cause of about one in every six deaths among diabetics who were under fifty years old when they died.

How do I know that I am getting ketoacidotic? For most people the first stage is a persistently high blood glucose level, usually associated with an infection or some other illness. You can test for ketones in the urine yourself. Buy the ketone testing sticks or get them from your doctor. If you cannot get your glucose level down within twenty-four to forty-eight hours by increasing your insulin and you have a lot of ketones in the urine, call your diabetic adviser.

If this happens when your usual doctor is away, remember that another doctor may be less familiar with your diabetes than your own so you will

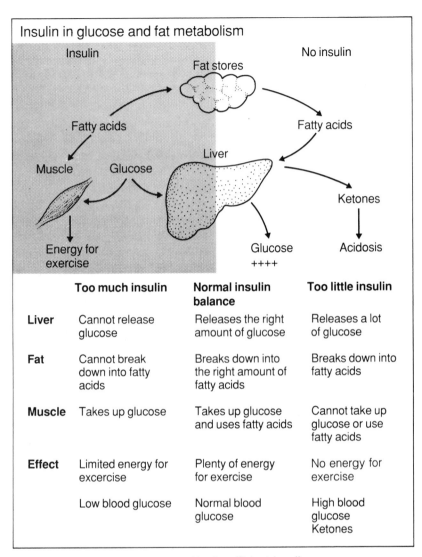

Insulin in glucose and fat metabolism

	Too much insulin	Normal insulin balance	Too little insulin
Liver	Cannot release glucose	Releases the right amount of glucose	Releases a lot of glucose
Fat	Cannot break down into fatty acids	Breaks down into the right amount of fatty acids	Breaks down into fatty acids
Muscle	Takes up glucose	Takes up glucose and uses fatty acids	Cannot take up glucose or use fatty acids
Effect	Limited energy for excercise	Plenty of energy for exercise	No energy for exercise
	Low blood glucose	Normal blood glucose	High blood glucose Ketones

The formation of ketones is caused by insufficient insulin.

need to do some explaining. If you know that things have really got out of hand and you have ketones in the urine or symptoms of ketosis, insist on going to the hospital.

Starvation ketosis Less frequently, people with diabetes develop starvation ketosis. Your blood glucose level may be low or high and you have lots of ketones because you have not been able to eat enough, for instance, during an illness when you vomited. Again, if you are not managing to eat very much and feeling ill, it is worth checking for ketones.

The risk of ketoacidosis is the reason why you must never stop your insulin.

Hospital treatment   When you are in the hospital, ketoacidosis is treated by infusing plenty of saline (salty water) with potassium into a vein. Treatment also includes either continuous intravenous insulin infusion or hourly intramuscular insulin injections. Your blood acid levels, glucose and potassium will be checked frequently. The infection or other illness which caused the ketoacidosis will be treated. You may be admitted to the intensive care unit so that a close eye can be kept on you. You should feel much better within a couple of days.

Ketone testing   It is useful to have a ketone testing kit in the house, but do not become obsessed with ketones. Virtually all insulin-treated diabetics show ketones occasionally. These usually settle with adjustments in diet or insulin. The time to worry is if you are showing a lot of ketones in every urine specimen.

The dawn phenomenon

Many people with diabetes have a sharp rise in their blood glucose just before they wake up in the morning. There is still some argument about precisely why this is, but many researchers believe that it is simply because blood insulin levels are getting lower. However, earlier in the night, your blood glucose may have been low, even hypoglycaemic. If you are waking with high blood glucose levels, check what is happening to your blood glucose during the night. Use an alarm clock to wake yourself up at, say, two and five in the morning to check your blood glucose level. Managing high pre-breakfast glucose levels depends on the type of insulin you are taking and whether you also have nocturnal hypoglycaemia.

High all the night   If you are running high throughout the night, the solution should be straightforward. Increase your long-acting or medium-acting evening insulin or, if you are overweight, eat a little less before you go to bed. If you are on a very long-acting insulin, taken only in the mornings, you may have to increase it, and then you may have to readjust your diet so that you do not go low in the afternoon or evening. If you have a late main evening meal, after about eight o'clock, you may need to increase your evening short-acting insulin, rather than the long-acting one.

51

Low then high It is a little more difficult to sort things out if you are hypoglycaemic during the night and you then awaken with a high blood glucose level. Obviously, if you increase your long-acting insulin, you may become seriously hypoglycaemic at two or three in the morning, before the insulin runs out. One way of coping is to have a rapidly absorbed snack just before you go to bed, rather than a very high fibre one from which the glucose is absorbed more slowly. This can be combined with a slight increase in your evening medium-acting or long-acting insulin and a slight decrease in your fast-acting insulin. Altering the quantity and timing of your main evening meal may help, if this is practical, and altering the time at which you give your insulin injection can also help sometimes. Discuss this with your doctor. If you cannot get it right on twice-daily insulin injections, consider splitting the evening injection so that you have the short-acting insulin before the main evening meal and the long-acting or medium-acting insulin before going to bed. Another approach is to try a CSII pump, which will give a constant insulin infusion throughout the night. Some models also allow you to program for delayed insulin boosts to cope with an early morning rise (for example, the CPI 9100 model).

People with insulin-treated diabetes should always eat a snack before going to bed.

Oral hypoglycaemic drugs

If you are taking oral hypoglycaemic pills and your blood or urine glucose levels become very high, consider increasing your dose. Naturally, whether you can do this depends on whether you are already on the maximum dose or not. If you are not on the maximum dose, try taking another half pill a day, or another whole pill if this does not take you over the maximum.

One of the problems of being on pills is that they may not be absorbed if you have diarrhoea or vomiting. Even if they are, they may not be sufficient to overcome the increased insulin resistance that can result from infection and other illnesses. If you have diarrhoea and vomiting or if you cannot bring your blood glucose level down yourself, or if you feel very ill, contact your doctor immediately. Sometimes it may be necessary to have insulin injections to control your blood glucose level during a time of illness. This does not necessarily mean that the insulin will need to be continued when you have recovered.

Loss of glucose control on oral hypoglycaemics

Many people with the form of diabetes that starts during middle age and the later years (maturity onset type) can control their blood glucose on diet and oral hypoglycaemic treatment. Most people whose diabetes begins under the age of thirty years need insulin treatment but a few with maturity onset diabetes of youth (MODY) can be treated successfully with oral agents. Control of your weight through diet is especially important in maturity onset diabetes because obesity increases the body's resistance to the action of insulin. However, if insulin production fails, whether in maturity onset diabetes or MODY, insulin injections will be needed for glucose control. This is not a disaster.

Geoffrey, who is now fifty-eight years old and a production manager, had been taking chlorpropamide since his diabetes was diagnosed five years previously, gradually increasing the dose to the maximum of 500 mg daily.

Despite sticking carefully to his diet and remaining at the ideal weight for his age and height, his glucose levels began to rise. His doctor added metformin treatment and the dose of this was increased to its maximum, but to no avail. Geoffrey's blood glucose levels continued to rise and he began to feel thirsty and had to get up to urinate several times each night. He felt tired and listless. I told him that he now needed insulin treatment but Geoffrey had a horror of injections and was convinced that he would never be able either to give his own insulin or allow anyone else to give it to him.

'I would sooner die than go on to insulin,' he said.

Nothing I said could persuade him to change his mind. Over the succeeding weeks he became increasingly ill, was drinking large quantities of fluids daily, started to lose weight and was irritable with his wife and family. He developed an embarrassing soreness around his penis, a fungal condition called thrush, which men and women with diabetes can develop with poor glucose control. This was treated but it recurred. At each clinic visit I tried to persuade Geoffrey to change his mind about insulin treatment but he remained adamant. Then finally one day he came into the clinic in tears. He could no longer do his job properly, he felt awful and was badly depressed. His wife, who came with him, was very worried about him. I got out an insulin syringe and needle and demonstrated on myself how simple it is to insert the needle under the skin. After thirty minutes' persuasion by me and his wife, Geoffrey stuck the needle into his arm.

'It doesn't hurt,' he said, astonished.

He is now on twice daily insulin injections with good glucose control, is back at work and says he feels marvellous. He wishes he had tried insulin sooner.

Call for help

Even the best informed and most efficient people have occasional problems. It is not an admission of defeat to call for help – just common sense. Doctors greatly prefer being called when they can help prevent a problem from getting worse than when a disaster has occurred. Contact your doctor sooner rather than later.

Problems with glucose control

- Hypoglycaemia is preventable. Learn your warning signs – and learn from your mistakes.
- Measure blood glucose levels frequently when you are ill.
- Plan what to do if you become ill before it happens.
- Take more insulin if your blood glucose level rises.
- Check for ketones if your blood glucose level rises or you cannot eat.
- Never stop taking your insulin.
- Do not be afraid to call for help.

4 How diabetes affects your body

Over the years, diabetes can cause damage to some body tissues. This is not inevitable and careful attention to blood glucose control may help you prevent it. The main tissues that can be affected are the eyes, nerves, kidneys, heart and blood vessels.

Eyes

Diabetic retinopathy is a condition in which the small blood vessels supplying the light-sensitive retina at the back of the eye become damaged. Eventually they can no longer supply nutrients and the starved retina releases an unknown factor which encourages proliferation of new vessels. Unfortunately these grow forwards away from the retina into the clear jelly or vitreous through which we see. The new vessels can tear and bleed into the vitreous, obstructing vision.

Such severe proliferative retinopathy is uncommon. Generally the only sign that the diabetic process is affecting the eye is what is called microaneurysm formation, when tiny red dots can be seen on or near the damaged blood vessels. These very early changes can be seen through an ophthalmoscope (a magnifying torch shone through the pupil of the eye) and warn of the development of retinopathy. Microaneurysms do not affect vision, but haemorrhages and fatty deposits (exudates) may also start to form on the retina. If these exudates lie over the area of best vision, which is called the macula (see the diagram opposite), sight may be impaired.

Diabetic retinopathy
1. Can be detected at an early stage
2. Can be treated successfully
3. May be prevented by careful attention to glucose control.

Eye checks Everyone with diabetes should have regular, preferably annual, visual acuity and retina checks. Your retina can be examined either with an ophthalmoscope after dilating drops have been put into your eye (the effects of these can be reversed after the examination) or with a special infra-red camera. The retinal camera produces a Polaroid picture within a few minutes, and because it uses infra-red light no dilating drops are needed.

If minor changes are found, all that is needed is a reassessment of your glucose balance and more frequent checks. If you have more severe changes, laser treatment is used with the aim of encouraging regression of proliferative vessels and preventing further new vessels forming. Laser treatment is usually carried out by an ophthalmologist and may have to be repeated. Anyone on treatment with normal blood glucose levels is less likely to develop retinopathy than people with high glucose levels. Lesions (microaneurysms, haemorrhages or exudates) may also regress if control is improved after retinopathy has developed, though it is obviously better to try to prevent them from appearing in the first place.

Cataracts These are more common among people with diabetes than in the general population. They are caused by deposits in the lens of

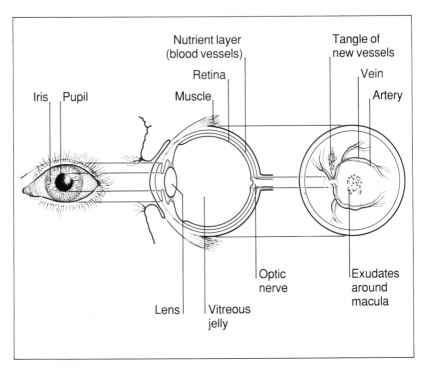

Left, a vertical section through a normal eye, and *right*, what the doctor sees when he looks through the pupil of someone with severe diabetic retinopathy.

the eye which block vision. They can be treated by removal of the eye's lens, which has become opaque. This is replaced either with an implanted lens, or you are given contact lenses or glasses. The operation has an excellent success rate. If you have diabetic retinopathy as well as cataracts, your ophthalmologist may have to treat the cataract before the extent of the retinopathy can be seen. Nowadays it can sometimes be removed as a day-case procedure.

See your doctor If you notice any change in your vision, see your doctor at once. Although cataracts and diabetic retinopathy may be the reason for a change in your vision, the most common cause is a high blood glucose level or a changing blood glucose level. This alters the focusing properties of the lens temporarily, causing blurring. The blurring disappears once your blood glucose level is controlled, so do not waste money on new glasses until you are sure that any change in your vision is not caused by glucose problems. Always bear these points in mind:

1. Tell your doctor immediately if your vision deteriorates.
2. The commonest cause of visual change in diabetes is high or changing glucose levels. Do not buy new spectacles when your glucose control is poor.
3. Regular eye checks can detect diabetic retinopathy at an early stage.
4. Diabetic retinopathy is treatable.
5. Diabetic retinopathy may be prevented by good glucose control.
6. People with diabetes may develop cataracts: they too can be treated.

Nerves

Many newly diagnosed diabetics notice tingling or pins and needles in their hands or feet. This is caused by an alteration of the function of the nerves supplying sensation to the hands or feet and tends to improve when the blood glucose is under control. Sometimes interference with nerve function lasts for longer, or develops several years after the diagnosis of diabetes. This is called neuropathy. Occasionally neuropathy may affect just one nerve or the working of the muscles instead of, or as well as, sensation. After many years of diabetes it is not unusual to have slight numbness of the feet. This is usually not unpleasant or very obvious but it means that you may not be aware of small rubs or cuts on your feet. If you do have numb feet you should get into the habit of looking at your feet every day so that you discover any small injuries and can protect them. Do not walk barefoot and ensure that your shoes cannot possibly rub.

Check for neuropathy You can find out if your feet are numb by yourself,

57

but your doctor can make more detailed checks. It is important that sensation is checked regularly so that small changes can be detected early. Vitamin deficiences are another cause of neuropathy that can be put right easily. Your doctor will be able to look for these.

As with retinopathy, studies have shown that people with diabetes who have neuropathy have had higher blood glucose levels in the preceding years than those who have not developed this complication. Furthermore, the symptoms of neuropathy may be improved with the return of the blood glucose level to normal. Occasionally a change to insulin treatment, even if your blood glucose control is all right, may produce an improvement in troublesome neuropathic symptoms. We do not fully understand why this works. There are also drugs that can be used to treat tingling or unusual sensations if these become unpleasant.

Autonomic neuropathy   This is a form of nerve damage that affects the nerves controlling such functions as blood pressure, erection of the penis, bowel action and bladder emptying. Autonomic neuropathy is not usually noticed by the person with diabetes; it causes no problems and is detected only by sophisticated testing. Just occasionally it does cause sufficient disturbance of these functions to be noticed:

- Postural hypotension: poor blood pressure control may cause postural hypotension, which is a fall in blood pressure on standing. This may make you feel dizzy when you get up from a chair or bed. Wearing supportive stockings to prevent pooling of blood in the legs may help. Drugs such as fludrocortisone may reduce the pressure drop.
- Diabetic bowel and bladder: autonomic neuropathy which involves the bowel may cause diarrhoea, and this may be especially troublesome at night. It can settle by itself. If not, the diarrhoea may improve with tetracycline (antibiotic) treatment.
  Incomplete emptying of the bladder is another effect, and occasionally leads to urinary tract infection in the urine that is not lost. Playing special attention to bladder emptying may improve this problem.
- Impotence caused by autonomic failure of erection is discussed in Chapter 6.

Loss of hypoglycaemic warnings   One practical problem for insulin-treated diabetics thought to be due to autonomic neuropathy is the reduction or loss of the warning symptoms of hypoglycaemia. This does not necessarily apply to everyone with autonomic neuropathy; on the other hand, over the years the warning of hypoglycaemia may be harder to recognize in people with no other signs of autonomic neuropathy.

Bear these points always in mind:

1. Transient tingling of the hands or feet is common before diabetes is diagnosed and usually settles with treatment.
2. Tingling or numbness in the feet may develop over the years.
3. If you have numb feet, examine them every night for minor injuries. Do not walk barefoot. Choose your shoes carefully.
4. Have regular check-ups for neuropathy.
5. Good glucose control may prevent the development of neuropathy, and improve it if symptoms have become apparent.
6. Symptomatic autonomic neuropathy is uncommon and many of its features are treatable.

Kidneys and urinary tract

I have already discussed retinopathy, a form of small blood vessel damage (the technical term is microangiopathy). Another tissue in which small vessels may be damaged is the kidney. In the kidney, urine is formed from waste substances and water that are passed from millions of tiny blood vessels into the drainage tubes. With diabetes, the walls of these blood vessels sometimes thicken until the waste substances and water can no longer pass out of the blood vessels to start forming urine. The kidneys have an enormous reserve capacity and most of the blood vessels have to be damaged before there is any noticeable effect.

Proteinuria The earliest sign of kidney damage is protein in the urine, called proteinuria. This can be discovered with urine tests and everyone with diabetes should have his or her urine checked for protein at regular intervals. Nowadays, many clinics are testing urine for microalbuminuria, tiny amounts of protein which may indicate the earliest stages of diabetic kidney damage in people with insulin-dependent diabetes. In those with non-insulin dependent diabetes microalbuminuria may indicate an increased risk of heart or other blood vessel problems. If it is found in several samples but without urinary tract infection (see below) other kidney tests can be carried out. Proteinuria does not necessarily mean you have other kidney function problems but it does indicate the need to check for them. If you have high blood pressure it must be very carefully controlled and frequent checks must be made for urinary tract infection.

Cystitis The commonest cause of proteinuria among people with diabetes is urinary tract infection, such as cystitis or bladder infection, pyelonephritis or kidney infection. A midstream urine sample is easily taken and will be sent to the laboratory for analysis so that appropriate antibiotics can be given. Non-diabetic men rarely have urinary tract infection but diabetic men may do so and it is common in women. The

59

symptoms are a burning sensation on passing urine which may have blood in it or smell bad, and a very frequent desire to pass urine, although there may be little there to pass. Urinary tract infection may upset your glucose balance and so your blood glucose levels should be checked frequently.

Thrush

One of the commonest early symptoms of diabetes among women is itching and soreness between the legs. The vulva and vaginal area, and sometimes the skin around the anus, are extremely sore and red and so itchy that the sufferer has a desperate desire to scratch, which is embarrassing and makes everything more sore. There is frequently a creamy vaginal discharge and the skin may be covered with white flecks. This condition is caused by the fungus which also produces thrush in babies. It can be cured by an antifungal cream (it is important to insert the cream high into the vagina to destroy the fungus completely) or by pessaries or special tampons. It is also important to control your blood glucose level, because the fungus likes a sugary environment.

Men can get thrush too (see also page 80), and may develop soreness of the penis. Thrush can be passed on by sexual intercourse and so both partners should use the antifungal cream.

The thrush fungus and other organisms may also colonize skin folds of very overweight people in places such as the groin, under the breasts and sometimes the umbilicus or belly button. This is because sweat collects there and provides a moist environment for the fungus to grow. Again, antifungal creams usually cure this, but the ultimate solution is to lose weight and to control your blood glucose level.

Heart and blood vessels

I have already described microangiopathy, a form of small blood vessel damage which may occur in diabetes. Large blood vessels can also be damaged in diabetes and this is called macroangiopathy (macro – large, angiopathy – blood vessel abnormality). Macroangiopathy is atherosclerosis, or hardening of large arteries. It is more common in diabetics than non-diabetics. Hard deposits of fatty tissue in the lining of the blood vessel obstruct and eventually block blood flow, or encourage blood clots to form on their roughened surfaces.

Intermittent claudication and angina Atherosclerosis may cause poor circulation in the legs, producing a cramp-like pain in the calves on walking, which is relieved by rest. This causes intermittent limping – the medical term is intermittent claudication.

If you suffer from this, check your feet daily so that small rubs or injuries can be treated immediately: poor circulation leads to poor healing. Do not let your feet get cold in winter; even in a temperate climate it is possible to get frostbite in winter if you have poor circulation. Atherosclerosis in the coronary arteries which supply the heart muscle may produce chest pain. This is because the muscle is not getting enough oxygen. This chest pain sometimes spreads down the left arm, and it is felt during exercise. It is called angina. If the blood supply to a particular area of heart muscle is completely blocked off, that muscle is damaged and a heart attack, or myocardial infarct, results.

Preventing the development of atherosclerosis
Smoking is a definite cause of atherosclerosis. There is no argument about this in medical and scientific circles. Smoking is bad for everyone, but especially for people with diabetes. If you are a smoker, stop now. Smoking is so dangerous that you should stop even at the expense of a temporary gain in weight, although obviously it is better not to gain weight if possible. If you are a non-smoker, do not start smoking.

Blood fats   Although elevation of the blood glucose is the most obvious abnormality in your body chemistry, fat metabolism is also affected. This may have the effect of raising your blood fat levels and making the development of arteriosclerosis more likely. It is therefore particularly important that anyone with diabetes does not eat excessive amounts of fat. Most researchers also think that the fat that diabetics eat should be low in saturated fats and high in polyunsaturates, but a few feel that this point is still debatable. As well as reducing fat, keeping to a high fibre diet is helpful in preventing the development of atherosclerosis.

Hypertension   High blood pressure of hypertension is more common among diabetics than non-diabetics. Various effects of diabetes, including atherosclerosis, contribute to this. The important message is that you should have your blood pressure checked at least once a year. If it is high it should be treated, because high blood pressure can put a strain on the heart and also lead to kidney damage and strokes. It may also add to the effects of diabetic angiopathy (see page 59).

If your doctor starts giving you treatment for hypertension, you must continue to take the pills for ever, or until the doctor tells you to stop. There are many different pills for the treatment of hypertension. If those you are taking do not agree with you, do not just stop taking them, but tell your doctor so that he or she can choose another drug that may suit you better.

Beta-blocking drugs (for example, propranolol, atenolol, metoprolol and other -olols) may reduce or suppress the warning signs of hypoglycaemia. This effect is more frequent with so-called non-selective or more widely active beta-blockers. Thiazide drugs (for example, bendrofluazide) may increase the blood glucose level and sometimes make mild, previously undetected, diabetes obvious. Thiazides cause diuresis or urinary water loss. Other diuretic drugs may be used to treat hypertension and can also increase the blood glucose level (for example, frusemide or bumetanide). Diuretic drugs cause sodium and potassium loss in the urine. Chlorpropamide can also produce a low blood sodium level and this may occasionally cause symptoms.

Many doctors advise people with hypertension to avoid added salt in their diet. There is still some controversy over this but it seems sensible to avoid excess salt. The food we eat contains what we need before flavouring is added.

Obesity　Being fat makes high blood pressure worse and also places a strain on your heart. It makes your cells resistant to the action of insulin. The solution is obvious.

Exercise　Exercise is discussed in Chapter 9. Regular exercise is also good for the circulation and the heart and helps keep your body sensitive to the effects of insulin. If you have poor circulation in the legs, regular exercise of the leg muscles, such as walking, helps alternative circulation to develop and improves the blood supply.

Always bear these points in mind:

1. Hardening of the arteries or atherosclerosis is more common in diabetics than in non-diabetics.
2. Atherosclerosis can cause poor circulation in the legs, coronary artery disease (angina, heart attacks), high blood pressure and strokes.
3. Much can be done to prevent atherosclerosis.
4. If you smoke stop. If you do not smoke – do not start.
5. Reduce your intake of fats. It is probably better to eat poly-unsaturated rather than saturated fats.
6. Eat a high fibre diet.
7. Avoid added salt.
8. Watch your blood pressure.
9. Do not get fat.
10. Exercise regularly.

Joints

Most people with diabetes do not realize that their joints may be affected. This condition is not often a nuisance, and most people do not even notice that they have it. What usually happens is that the tendons and ligaments of the hands get a bit tight and, for example, you cannot flatten all your fingers against the table with your hand palm down. This condition goes under the wonderful name of cheiroarthropathy. If your hands are getting a bit stiff, get into the habit of doing a few finger exercises every day, perhaps with your hands in warm water. Playing an imaginary piano, clenching and straightening your fist and stretching your fingers as straight as they will go are useful exercises.

Very rarely, people with bad neuropathy get a severe form of joint trouble called Charcot's joints. This is usually in the feet or ankles and may develop after a minor injury. If you have bad neuropathy and have a sprained ankle or foot injury which does not improve, insist on repeated x-rays.

Feet

Because our feet are so far away from the rest of us, there is a tendency to forget about them. But if you have diabetes you must look after your feet as carefully as you do your face.

Mavis closed the front door and staggered into the sitting room with her shopping. She collapsed onto the sofa and pulled off her new shoes. "My feet are killing me," she gasped as she put them up and reached for a cigarette.

Two weeks later, her feet were killing her. The blisters from her new shoes had become infected, the infection had spread up her legs and she had developed septicaemia (blood poisoning). Fortunately, good control of her diabetes and large doses of antibiotics saved her life. An operation to bypass her blocked atherosclerotic leg arteries and restore her circulation saved her legs. Her husband threw away her cigarettes and her new shoes.

Diabetes causes circulatory problems and the arteries which supply the feet can become furred up (atherosclerotic). Diabetic nerve damage often affects the feet causing numbness. This means that you may not realise that you have injured or rubbed your foot, or that your shoes do not fit. If you have joint problems in the feet or other reasons for your foot to rub on your shoe or abnormal pressure areas to develop, ulcers can occur at the pressure sites. If your blood glucose is high your body cannot fight infection as well as it should. All these factors combine to cause ulcers, gangrene and infections. In the most severe cases the only solution may be amputation of the foot or leg.

Foot care is a part of basic diabetes self-care. Keep your feet clean and wear socks/tights which cannot rub inside shoes which fit comfortably from the start. Trim the nails straight across, smoothing the corners so that they cannot dig in. Check your feet every night and seek help immediately if you notice anything wrong. Most problems are minor and can be treated rapidly. Neglected minor problems are what cause major problems. Be especially vigilant on holiday.

I'm frightened

There is no need to be. If you are aware of the risks, you can take preventive action before these conditions have a chance to develop. If you have regular check-ups, minor changes can be identified at a time when something can be done about them. This is one reason why it is important to keep your appointments even if you feel well and your blood glucose levels are all right. Most people with diabetes are untroubled by complications, and even if you develop them, a great deal can be done to treat them.

- Have regular health check-ups.
- Tell your doctor at once if you have any trouble with your vision; notice any change in sensation in your limbs; have pain or burning on passing urine or need to urinate very often; have soreness or irritation between the legs; pain in your calves when you walk; pain in your chest; or any problems with your feet.
- Do not smoke.
- Watch your weight.
- Eat a high fibre diet, without added salt, with reduced fat content, low in saturated and high in polyunsaturated fats.
- Keep your blood glucose levels normal.
- Take any pills prescribed by your doctor.

5 School and growing up

Most people with insulin-treated diabetes first learn that they have diabetes while they are school-children. Most people with maturity onset diabetes discover their diabetes when they are working or after they have retired. Whether you are sixteen or sixty years old, the news that you have diabetes comes as a shock. It is important to get back to your usual daily routine as quickly as possible and thereafter not to allow your diabetes to get in your way. Being diabetic should not prevent you from achieving what you want from life, whether it is a senior management position, a holiday in the sun, a job as a sales assistant or a college education.

School

Adjusting food and insulin Life at school usually has a regular pattern and times of energy output (whether mental or physical) are predictable. This means that you can adjust your food and insulin pattern to suit your activities with a reasonable amount of accuracy.

It is probably easier to take a constant dose of insulin and alter your food intake according to what you will be doing next. However, if you have a very energetic morning or afternoon on the same day every week, it may be helpful to reduce your insulin on that day. For example, you could reduce short-acting for morning activity and intermediate-acting for the afternoon in addition to eating more.

Tom is fourteen years old and takes twelve units of Actrapid (short-acting insulin) and twenty units of Monotard (long-acting insulin) in the morning before breakfast and eight units of Actrapid before his main evening meal. On Tuesdays he has history and geography before break-time, woodwork until lunch-time and football all afternoon.

He has had a couple of mild hypoglycaemic episodes during football in the past, so he reduces his Monotard insulin to seventeen units on Tuesday mornings, but still takes twelve units of Actrapid. He has his normal breakfast but eats an extra apple at break-time if he is going to do a lot of sawing in woodwork. At lunch-time he has an extra helping of potato and a double portion of dessert. Half-way through football he has a chocolate bar and an apple. He also has a couple of biscuits or crackers before he changes after the lesson, because he will be riding his bicycle home. On some Tuesdays he checks his blood glucose level several times during the day to see if his dietary and insulin changes are being successful.

Teaching teachers Children spend nearly half their waking hours at school and school heads and teachers should be told that a pupil has diabetes. Teachers should be given:

1. Precise details of the pupil's dietary and treatment needs.
2. Clear instructions as to what to do should problems arise.

The British Diabetic association provides information folders for parents to give to schools. Most diabetic clinics are also happy to help in this way. It is important that every teacher who comes into contact with your child is taught about diabetes. This may mean speaking to fifteen to twenty teachers – and repeating the discussion each year as your child moves up in the school. Informing the teachers can be organized more efficiently through the principal. It also helps if your child's classmates know about his or her diabetes, so that they understand why the extra food and injections are needed.

Janine is fifteen years old and has been diabetic for three years. For about a year her diabetes was very difficult to control. At that time she would have severe hypoglycaemic episodes of which she had no warning. It was not unusual for her suddenly to fall to the ground unconscious, a very rare problem for people with diabetes. Her best friend at school, Sue, knew nothing about diabetes until she met Janine. Now Sue has learned to recognize an impending hypoglycaemic attack and gives her friend glucose immediately.

During the bad year, Sue also calmly dealt with the more severe episodes, awakening Janine from coma by rubbing glucose tablets inside her mouth. She came to think of coping with Janine's attacks as part of her daily routine and neither she nor their other school-friends were unduly disturbed by them.

Fortunately these bad hypoglycaemic attacks stopped and Janine's diabetes is now better controlled.

Examinations and reviews

School reviews, whatever the pupil's age, are always times of stress. Examinations may determine the future; higher education colleges and universities and many employers use examination grades as a criterion for choosing candidates for interview. It is therefore vitally important that the diabetic pupil:

1. Does not miss classes because of his diabetes
2. Is able to concentrate during class
3. Devotes the necessary time to homework and studying for exams
4. Performs at his best during the review.

Do not miss classes Careful monitoring of the diabetes and rapidly sorting out any problems, particularly the blood glucose level during coughs and colds, should minimize the time spent away from school. You should be able to concentrate well if your blood glucose level is normal, whereas very high or low blood glucose levels may cause muddled thinking.

Studying for exams This inevitably involves a lot of sitting and reading with little energy output. Coupled with increasing stress as the examination approaches, this tends to raise the blood glucose level. This may become worse if you 'worry eat' while working – many small nibbles soon add up. Your normal diet may need to be decreased and low calorie snacks added. Resist the temptation to allow your blood glucose level to run high 'just until the exam is over'. Your brain may not be working as efficiently as it should if the blood glucose level is high. If you take up an academic career there will be many examinations to come, so you must get used to taking them in your stride.

Some people with diabetes find that their blood glucose levels fall when they are worrying about grades. It is therefore important to check the blood glucose to find out what is happening.

The day of the review On the day of the review it is essential that there is no risk of hypoglycaemia and also that your blood glucose is not very high. Make sure that the examiner is told in advance that you may need to check your blood glucose level before, during or after the review and that you must have food and drink available during the examination. It is sensible to run your blood glucose around 7 or 8 mmol/l (126 or 144 mg/dl) rather than 4 mmol/l (72 mg/dl). You should take your blood testing kit, cans or containers of fruit juice, biscuits or crackers, glucose tablets or candies and tissues into the assessment with you. Make sure that you check your blood glucose before you go into the examination, and eat something if it is low. If you do, wipe your fingers – a sticky paper could lose you marks! Do not panic if your blood glucose level is higher than you would like – it

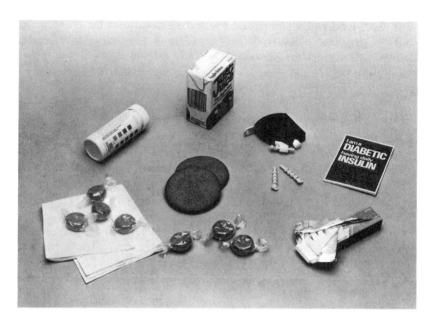

Diabetic kit to take into an examination: blood testing kit to check glucose before the examination starts, paper tissues, fruit juice, biscuits or cookies, glucose tablets, glucose sweets or candies and your diabetic card.

is not a disaster and you will not fail because of it! Just think afterwards what you could have done to achieve better glucose control so that you can learn for the next time.

School trips

In the old days pupils with diabetes were sometimes left behind when the rest of the class went off on a school trip because the teachers were afraid that they would not be able to cope if something went wrong. This made the diabetic pupils feel very left out. Nowadays they should be able to share in all class activities. There is no problem if you can measure your blood glucose level and adjust your own insulin and food, and if the supervisors are all told how to recognize and treat a hypoglycaemic episode.

For younger pupils or inexperienced diabetic teenagers, the teachers need to be given more information about coping with the diabetes. If parents are asked to help with the trip, your mother or father could come along. Supervisors may feel happier if they have a telephone number to call in an emergency, although few will have to use it.

Planning   The first thing to do on hearing of a school trip is to find out exactly what is planned and for how long you will be away. Then work out how much food you will need and add some extra snacks for extra energy and an extra meal in case of delays (see Chapter 11 on travel). Take your insulin and blood testing kit and some money. Of course, you will be carrying glucose tablets and some form of identity card, locket or bracelet.

Growing up

For everyone, being a teenager is an exciting and confusing time. It is a time when you start moving away from your parents and exploring life on your own. You want to do your own thing, and at the same time fit in with your friends – wear the right kind of clothes, eat the same, and stay out late at night. It can be very embarrassing being the odd one out. As a teenager, your parents always seem to be nagging you – clean your room, don't come home late, have you done your homework? So you rebel and then feel guilty because you love them really. The older generation just do not seem to understand you. You want to burst out into the world and do great things and suddenly it all seems very large and frightening and you feel rather lost.

Nowadays, the world can seem very unkind if you leave school ready to work, then find you cannot get a job. You start off applying for the exciting jobs, then the possible ones, then any jobs. Being turned down by prospective employers is no fun for anyone. Being unemployed is depressing and boring. If you have been lucky enough to get a job or go on to further education, this too has its good and bad moments. You want to do well and create a good impression and there is a lot to take in all at once. Your safe circle of school-friends have moved on and you have to start making new friends.

Parental worries

What I have just said can apply to any teenager. It may seem much harder if you are a diabetic teenager. For a start you have to be a little more organized than your friends. You have to take your insulin injections once or twice a day and you have to eat meals at about the same time each day which have the right food content. You cannot just go out to a disco and dance the night away on two beers and some potato chips. Everyone with diabetes gets fed up about their disorder at times. 'Why me? Why have I been singled out in this way? It is not fair.' 'Why should I take my insulin anyway? I'm not going to take it today – so there!' But the only person you are fighting in the long run is yourself, and it is no fun waging war on your own body. So you get frustrated instead and get depressed, or get angry with your parents or friends. No one expects you to be perfect; there is no such person as a perfect diabetic. It is natural to resent being diabetic at times, so do not feel guilty about it.

The parents of someone with diabetes can be a little more worried about their teenage son or daughter than other people's parents. Their concern may come across as extra nagging. Have you had your insulin? Have you checked your blood glucose? You must be home for supper. Why were you late home last night? We were worried, we thought you might have had a hypoglycaemic attack. In the early teenage years, your mother or father may still be giving you your insulin injections and taking most of the responsibility for looking after your diabetes. Some parents find it very difficult to realize that you are now old enough to take over this responsibility for yourself.

Jane is now twenty years old and has been diabetic for ten years. When she was nineteen she went on the local diabetic association holiday and was thoroughly enjoying herself. She telephoned her mother to tell her all about the holiday. During the conversation her mother asked her about her diabetic control.

Later that night I had a telephone call from her mother, who said, among other things, 'Jane's blood glucose is 10 mmol/l (180 mg/dl). I am sure you are doing something about that!'

A single reading of 10 mmol/l is hardly a disaster, but the whole telephone conversation showed how over-anxious and over-protective Jane's mother was. Jane was a sensible and intelligent young woman and would have been mortified to learn that her mother had telephoned me. A year later, Jane succeeded in leaving home and now has a demanding and exciting job. She continues to look after her own diabetes efficiently.

Handing over responsibility
Parental concern is natural and it is very difficult and worrying to give up running your child's diabetes. There is the constant fear of hypolgycaemia and the unspoken dread of your child being found unconscious or ill in the street. The teenage years with their rebellions and new activities must seem to many parents the worst possible time to hand over the care of the diabetes to the teenager. But most doctors believe that the diabetic child should start learning to look after his or her own diabetes as soon as possible. Very small children can give their own insulin injections and by the time they have reached their teens all diabetics should be injecting themselves. Similarly, all diabetic children should learn to measure their own blood glucose level as soon as possible and should gradually start to make their own decisions about adjusting their insulin dose according to the results. If the handover process from parent to child is gradual it is easier on both sides; you should not forget that your child may be as frightened of taking over responsibility as you are of relinquishing it. During this time your child must learn the rules.

Steve became diabetic when he was eleven years old and was allowed to eat what he wanted as long as he ate enough to stop him from becoming hypoglycaemic. When he started going to an adult diabetic clinic in another city he was appalled to discover that his blood glucose control was poor and that he had been eating the wrong foods for years. He deeply regrets not having been encouraged to eat a sensible diet from the time his diabetes was diagnosed as it is very hard to change now. He feels let down and angry.

Enjoying life

How can a diabetic teenage enjoy life without the diabetes getting in the way? Your ticket to trouble-free fun is a little common sense and forward planning. First, make sure you are so practised at checking your blood glucose level that you can do it quickly and efficiently anywhere. Get all your blood testing kit into an easily portable form that will fit into a pocket or bag. If you can keep an eye on your blood glucose level you can allow yourself more flexibility over insulin injections and meal times.

Insulin On most occasions you will be able to take your morning insulin injection at home. There is no reason for you to come home to take your evening insulin. Draw it up in the morning and put the syringe in a small case or bag. Nowadays there are several devices such as BD Lilly pen or Novopen that can easily be carried in a pocket (see Chapter 2). Even an ordinary plastic syringe with needle, filled with insulin is reasonably portable, especially if you find a carrying case which prevents the plunger being pushed in by mistake. An empty syringe with needle and bottles of insulin with a foil-wrapped swab can also be carried in a pocket or case. You can then make a quick blood glucose check and give the appropriate insulin injection wherever you are.

Wendy has had diabetes for 14 of her 20 years. "She was always so good about her injections" said her mother, "and she always ate her diet and did her tests perfectly. Now I just can't do a thing with her. Out all hours, won't eat what I give her, eats junk food, not a single blood test this month. What are we to do with her, doctor?" Wendy sat in her bed looking at the wall. She had just recovered from an episode of diabetic ketoacidosis. "What do you think about your diabetes, Wendy?" I asked. "I'm fed up with it," she replied sullenly. "What makes you most fed up?" "Having to come home for my insulin."

During our discussion Wendy said that she felt her diabetes was stopping her from doing everything she wanted – getting a job, going out with her friends, eating nice food. Life was just not worth living. Wendy and her mother seemed to be fighting over the diabetes, yet Wendy was 20 years old. From what Wendy said, all anyone ever did about her diabetes was tell her off. When I told Wendy about insulin pens which would allow her freedom to go out, her mother developed a disapproving silence. But Wendy relaxed for the first time, and smiled a little, "Could I really have one of those?" she asked. "Of course," I said. She agreed to come to the Young Adult diabetic clinic.

Food Breakfast will usually be at home and should give you a good start to the day. One way of ensuring that you get the right type of lunch is to take a packed meal with you. There are several books that give a dietary breakdown of take-away foods. If this is the kind of meal you and your friends have, learn which of the items on the menu fit into your diet. A little dietary homework can reduce anxiety. Many sandwich shops now serve wholewheat bread and a wide variety of fillings and you can often buy baked potatoes with fillings. It will help if you carry an apple and some high fibre bars with you to fill in gaps and to use as snacks.

An evening out If you go out with your friends after school or work, eat a snack and find a quiet moment to check your blood glucose level. You can keep yourself going on snacks until everyone decides to have a meal. It is not a disaster if your evening meal is one or two hours late provided you stoke up with snacks and keep an eye on your blood glucose level. When the time comes for the main evening meal, take your insulin, remembering to adjust the dose according to your blood glucose level and what you plan to do afterwards. If you are going to a disco or ice skating rink or any other activity which will be energetic, take less short-acting insulin than you would usually have.

It is better to take your insulin somewhere clean than in a dirty lavatory. If you have told your friends that you have diabetes, there is no harm in taking it in front of them. They may be startled at first, but will almost certainly be interested in the insulin and diabetes. After a while, it will simply be a usual part of an outing and no one will bother if you just take out your insulin and syringe and give yourself the injection. If you treat the practical aspects of diabetes as ordinary and matter-of-fact, so will your friends. The abdomen is a useful place if you are taking your insulin in public because you can just undo your blouse or shirt and give yourself the injection. If you are sitting at a table very few people will notice what you are doing.

As the evening runs on you may need extra snacks to keep going, and you will certainly need something extra to eat if you are out at a time when you would usually be in bed.

Alcohol
Can people with diabetes drink alcohol? Yes, providing they stick to the rules. Alcohol blocks the release of glucose from the liver and can produce

hypoglycaemia in people with and without diabetes. It takes smaller amounts of alochol to produce this effect if you have diabetes requiring insulin than if you do not. Therefore, you must not have too much to drink at any one time. How much is too much? More than two pints of beer, or three US beers, or two short drinks. Always eat something if you have an alcoholic drink, such as some peanuts or nuts and raisins (these are available in most bars) or potato chips if there is nothing else, although they are too greasy to form a regular part of your diet.

Remember that alcohol is a calorie source (see p. 25) and must be counted as part of your diet. You must not count it as a carbohydrate exchange but just as part of the total calories. Remember too that low-carbohydrate beers and lagers have a higher alcohol content than ordinary beers. Do not be tempted to binge. Intersperse your alcoholic drinks with low-calorie soft drinks if you want to keep up with your friends. Getting drunk may seem like fun at the time but you may make yourself crashingly hypoglycaemic and no one will notice, least of all you!

Smoking
People with diabetes do not smoke. All the reasons for not smoking that apply to non-diabetics are equally valid for diabetics. Some are more so. People with diabetes are at greater risk of developing arteriosclerosis or hardening of the arteries than non-diabetics and smoking is a very good way of furring up your arteries (see also Chapter 4). In practical terms this can mean having a heart attack or getting such bad gangrene in your legs that they have to be amputated.

Yes, but that is a longterm problem. I'm interested in now! Fine. Smoking can make you ill now. Just smoking one cigarette can halve the rate at which insulin is absorbed. This is because the nicotine from the cigarette constricts blood vessels throughout your body. A diabetic smoker may have very irregular insulin absorption and very poor blood glucose control. Smokers need more insulin than non-smokers to control their diabetes.

Puberty and growth
This means the changes in hormone balance that change a child into an adult capable of producing children. These changes are one reason why teenagers start feeling different and why their moods may go up and down. As with non-diabetics, there is a wide range of ages at which signs of sexual development start to appear.

Girls As a rule, girls develop sexually at an earlier age than boys. Their breasts start to swell and the nipples and surrounding ring of tissue develop an adult shape. Hair grows over the pubic area and under the arms and menstrual periods start. For many diabetic women, period times are no different from any other part of the month, but for about a third, the build up to a period means a change in blood glucose control. Some women find that their insulin dose increases greatly before periods and suddenly falls after the bleeding starts. A few find that their control is unchanged until they start to bleed. Then they suddenly start going hypoglycaemic and need much less insulin for one or two days. Few girls have completely regular periods to start with and if you tend to have a rise in blood glucose around period time, you may find your glucose going up and down as your periods come and go. The only thing you have to do is make sure that you are on a flexible insulin pattern, for example, a very long-acting insulin with as many short-acting injections as you need, or twice daily short-acting and medium-acting insulins, and adjust things day-by-day. You may find that your moods go up and down too. It is not uncommon to feel grumpy or depressed before a period, and some women have fluid retention as well.

It is important to remember that you are capable of having babies as soon as your first period starts. The myth that all diabetic women are sterile is completely untrue, as several surprised diabetic mothers have found!

Boys As boys develop, changes occur in their body hair, voice and in the size of the penis and testes; wet dreams and morning erections occur which usually precede the ability to have a full erection on stimulation. These developments of manhood do not usually have a dramatic effect upon blood glucose control. What does change is the amount of food you need, and with it the dose of insulin. As you develop your full adult body size you need more and more food, and more insulin to help convert it into body tissue.

This increased fuel demand also affects girls, but to a lesser extent. But do not eat too much. Puppy fat does not just disappear; there is rarely any excuse for getting fat!

The hormonal changes which produce normal body growth are complex and are sensitive to chemical abnormalities in the body and other illnesses. Furthermore, the body has to be able to use all the glucose you gain from digesting your food. If your insulin balance is wrong and the glucose you need for growing is in the blood and cannot get into the tissues you will not grow normally. This can mean you end up much shorter than you should have done. Your body does not wait for your diabetic control to improve. Once you have missed your growth spurt you will stay short. So, eat the right amount for growing tall but not fat and keep your blood glucose levels normal to achieve your full potential.

Self-destruction

I have already discussed the need to rebel that most teenagers feel as they grow away from home and take a poke at authority. For some mixed-up teenagers, their diabetes provides the ideal weapon to get back at their parents, doctors and teachers. But, unfortunately, the only people they really harm are themselves. Every diabetic clinic has a small group of teenagers who are for ever in and out of the hospital in hypoglycaemic coma or ketoacidosis. They give themselves insulin overdoses or stop their insulin for days at a time. They are usually very good at judging exactly how much extra insulin to give or how little. But every so often, one of them gets it wrong. Instead of waking up to find Mum and Dad looking anxiously down at them, they die. Those who survive may have done themselves permanent harm. Many of the ketoacidosis experts have had so many intravenous drips that they no longer have any clear veins left into which life-saving drugs can be injected.

Very few self-destructive diabetics are quite as calculating as I have suggested. Some of them may be desperately trying to get across the message that they are very unhappy.

Martin was fourteen years old when I first met him. He had had diabetes for three years and for half of that time he had been in and out of hospital with extremely severe hypoglycaemia. On several occasions he had been unconscious for days at a time.

He went on a diabetic camp holiday and for the first three nights was severely hypoglycaemic every night. Then a member of the staff saw him injecting himself with ten times the amount of insulin he should have had. Martin knew he had been seen and for the next few nights his diabetic control yo-yo'd from very low to very high, ending up with an episode of diabetic ketoacidosis.

When he returned home he confessed that he had been overdosing with insulin for eighteen months. He had been doing it because he felt it was the only way he could express how much he hated having diabetes and having to inject himself every day. He is happier now that he can talk about his feelings and has stopped overdosing, although his glucose control is still not very good.

What many teenagers with diabetes do not realize is that doctors and others involved in looking after diabetes understand that being diabetic can seem an impossible burden at times. You can say anything you like to your doctor, he is not just there to tell you to eat the right things and measure your blood glucose and give you the right amount of insulin. We know that everyone with diabetes has times when their control is very far from perfect. Plenty of diabetics have forgotten to give themselves an insulin injection at the right time at some stage. No one can be perfect all the time. All we ask is that you try your best. If things are going wrong, tell us – perhaps we can help. If you are feeling fed up and frustrated, tell us. When you are seeing the doctor, however busy he seems, you have the right to talk about your problems. If you feel that you need more time to talk, ask for another appointment and explain why.

Many clinics have diabetic specialist nurses or other helpers. Some people find them less intimidating and easier to talk to than the doctor. If you really feel that you cannot talk about all your worries and fears to the doctor who looks after your diabetes, ask your family doctor if you can see someone else. Similarly, if your family doctor is really not on your wavelength, ask him if you can see another doctor. (I talk more about your relationship with your diabetic adviser in Chapter 12.)

College or university

Anna developed diabetes when she was eighteen years old, just three months before she was due to start at a university about a hundred miles from her home town. She had brilliant examination grades and a promising career lay ahead of her. When the time came to start university she refused to go. She said that she knew she would not be able to cope with her diabetes at the university. No amount of explanation and assurance could persuade her otherwise. She allowed her diabetes to destroy her future.

Anna's story is sadly not unique. For her, the combination of leaving home and coping with the practicalities of diabetes became overwhelming. But of course, the problem can easily be solved with a little common sense and care. I saw many diabetic students in Oxford thoroughly enjoying the academic and not-so-academic side of university life. Their diabetes is simply part of their everyday routine, rarely intruding on what they want to do.

Leaving home

For someone with diabetes, leaving home means moving away not only from your family but also from the doctors and other people who have been helping you to look after your diabetes, maybe since you were a child. Of course you can still see them during vacations, but what happens if you need help in term time? Most students register with the college doctor or with a local family doctor to cover them during term time. You can still see your own family doctor when you are at home. Most towns have a diabetic clinic. Ask your diabetic clinic doctor to contact the clinic in your college town and ask if the doctor there will keep an eye on you.

Of course, if you are moving to a new town permanently, your records will be transferred to your new family doctor and diabetic clinic. You will soon get used to the new team. Remember that different areas may do things a little differently. There is often more than one way of coping with a diabetic problem and there are several views on most aspects of care.

Always bear these points in mind:
- A diabetic pupil should not miss classes because of his or her diabetes.
- Control should be good enough for concentration in class as well as for homework and studying for exams. All diabetic pupils must be able to perform at their best during exams.
- All the student's teachers should know about his or her diabetes and what to do about hypoglycaemia.
- There is no reason why diabetics should not go on school trips.
- You should gradually take over the responsibility for your diabetes from your parents – and parents should start letting go.
- Feel free to go out with your friends and try new foods and new experiences. But use a little common sense; your parents were teenagers once and their advice is worth listening to.
- Drink alcohol in moderation if you want to but eat something with it.
- Do not smoke.
- Remember that as soon as diabetic girls have started menstruating and diabetic boys have erections, they are capable of creating children.
- If you leave home make sure that you arrange for a new family doctor and diabetic adviser to take over your care.
- Talk about your worries to your parents or to your doctor. Do not let your diabetes get you down. Go out and enjoy life.

6 Sex

Partnership

Every close relationship with a member of the opposite sex is a form of partnership, a sharing of experiences and ideas between two people. Some partnerships are short, others may last a lifetime. To start with you may be shy about telling your new partner that you have diabetes for fear that he or she will break off the relationship. But hiding your diabetes may lead to more and more lies and evasions. How do you explain that you have to eat within a certain time? If you are taking insulin, how do you manage to do it secretly? What happens if you have a hypoglycaemic attack?

Diana, a seventeen-year-old, met her boyfriend, John, at an ice skating rink. They both enjoyed skating and soon began spending every Tuesday evening together at the rink. One evening Diana had to work late at college and missed her evening meal. She thought that she had made up her carbohydrate intake with crackers and an apple but unfortunately she collapsed with a severe hypoglycaemic attack at the side of the rink. John was very frightened when he could not wake her up and the staff at the ice rink called an ambulance which rushed her to the hospital. No one knew that Diana had diabetes, but routine checks in the casualty department showed she had a low blood glucose level and she was soon revived.

John, much relieved, took her home. He was very upset that she had not trusted him enough to tell him about her diabetes – especially because his aunt was diabetic and he would have known what to do if he had realized that Diana was simply hypoglycaemic. They are still going out three years later.

Eventually you may both decide that you want to make your partnership permanent. By this time you should certainly have told your partner that you have diabetes and he or she should know what this means to you in practical terms, now and in the future. It is a good idea if your partner learns how to help you check on your diabetes and also about your diet and how to give you your insulin or pills.

Your diabetic adviser will be happy to see your partner with you and explain things if you wish. It is important that you have frank and open discussions about all aspects of your diabetes. It can also be helpful to discuss sex and families at this time.

Sex in relationships

Most people start to discover the pleasurable feelings of sexual excitement by exploring their own bodies. As you grow up you learn both to give and to receive sexual pleasure in close relationships with members of the opposite sex. Sexual contact may be confined to kissing and cuddling or may extend to full sexual intercourse. Sexual attraction may be a major reason for getting together or be only a small factor in your partnership. Whatever importance you give it within your relationship, remember that it is a shared experience and that you should both pay as much attention to giving pleasure as to receiving it. People with diabetes can gain as much pleasure from the sexual aspects of a relationship as anyone else.

Intercourse

Sexual intercourse is a pleasurable and important part of a close relationship for men and women. This applies to people with or without diabetes. The act of intercourse itself is a form of exercise and often happens at a time when you would usually be resting. If you are having intercourse regularly at night you may need to increase your bedtime snack or reduce your evening insulin, especially if you tend to have low glucose levels during the night. If you are an insulin-treated diabetic you should keep some glucose tablets under the pillow or beside the bed so that you can eat them quickly should you feel hypoglycaemic, for whatever reason. If you have intercourse at other times, perhaps unexpectedly, and you know that it will bring your glucose down, eat some food or a couple of glucose tablets immediately afterwards. An unexpected hypoglycaemic attack can spoil a beautiful relationship!

Sometimes, before your diabetes is controlled, or at times of poor glucose control, you may not feel much like sex because you are just not very fit. Indeed, you may feel below par generally and need as much sleep as you can get. You may be snappy or irritable with the people you love. As your glucose levels return towards normal, your energy levels should improve, and this includes your sexual energy and desire for intercourse. If your glucose is high you may not be a very relaxing person to share a bed with because the increased urine output makes you get up to pass urine during the night and you have to keep drinking because you are thirsty. Also, if you have soreness in the genital area from thrush, you may find intercourse uncomfortable. The accompanying discharge may be unattractive for your partner too. As described in Chapter 4, thrush can be treated simply and easily.

Impotence

One of the myths about diabetes is that all diabetic men are impotent. This is nonsense. Most diabetic men are normally potent but a few develop impotence in later years, and this is more common among men with diabetes than non-diabetics. If you think that you may be impotent, do not bottle your worries up inside you but discuss them with your doctor. He will not be embarrassed or think it odd that you want to discuss your sex life. If you go to a diabetes specialist he will probably also have trained in endocrinology or hormone disorders and be used to discussing such problems.

The impotence associated with diabetes is thought to be due to autonomic neuropathy (see page 58) because the autonomic nervous system is responsible for the increase in blood flow to the penis which causes it to become firm and erect. However, one study showed that two-thirds of diabetic men who were troubled by impotence were having wet dreams or morning erections. If this is the case, impotence during inter-course or masturbation is more likely to be due to psychological factors and may improve with counselling. One of the problems is that the more you worry about whether you are going to have an erection while making love, the more likely you are not to have one. If you and your partner can relax about this aspect of love making and not aim for full intercourse for a few weeks or months, but enjoy each other in different ways, things may improve. Many hospitals have counselling services for people with sexual problems. It is important to share your worries with your partner. She will then be able to help you as well.

But what if you are having no erections at all? The first thing to do is to have a full medical check-up. It may be that there is a non-diabetic hormonal reason for your impotence that can be put right by hormone injections. Your doctor will certainly want to take some blood tests to check this. Many illnesses, including uncontrolled diabetes, are associated with temporary impotence and loss of sexual drive. Full potency may return if the illness is treated and sometimes returns if the blood glucose is brought back under control, although this does not always happen.

If after a lot of tests your doctor tells you that you have impotence due to autonomic neuropathy, do not despair. It may be that you and your partner have the sort of relationship in which the sexual act plays only a small part. It is very important that you discuss things fully with your partner. She may be less upset than you imagine and there are other ways of giving each other pleasure. There are several treatments to help impotence. Injections of papaverine into the penis produce an erection in most cases and you can find the dose which suits you. Rarely this causes a prolonged erection which can be painful. There are several sheath-like devices which produce an erection by inducing a vacuum around the penis. Some men prefer penile implants – unlike the other methods these are permanent. Hormone injections are no use for neuropathic impotence; they simply increase the desire without improving the performance.

Contraception
Diabetic girls are capable of having babies as soon as they start having menstrual periods, and diabetic boys can father children once they are able to have an erection and ejaculate. Therefore, it is important that you take as much care to prevent unwanted pregnancies as a non-diabetic person. Methods of contraception are described below. The figures given for failure rates are approximate and apply to couples who are using the method properly. They are calculated as the number of women who become pregnant out of a hundred women using that method for a year. The failure rates are much higher if you include all couples using a particular method, because many people do not follow the instructions carefully.

Rhythm method This relies on the safe period, the time between menstrual bleeding and ovulation. It works only for women with absolutely regular periods, and even then is not wholly reliable. The rhythm method is not an efficient form of contraception. At least fifteen out of 100 women using it for a year will become pregnant.

If measuring your temperature is used to discover when ovulation has occurred, it is slightly more effective. Then the failure rate is five pregancies per 100 women a year.

This method is not recommended unless you have very strong religious or moral reasons for avoiding a more effective method.

Withdrawal This is completely unreliable. The idea is that the man withdraws his penis from the vagina before ejaculation so that no sperm enter the vagina. However, sperm can leak from the penis before full ejaculation takes place. It may also be very difficult for the man to withdraw at the critical moment. Furthermore, you should remember that it is possible for sperm to enter the vagina even without full penetration taking place. If you are indulging in heavy petting and there is any contact between the penis and the female genitalia, you need full contraceptive protection.

Sheath The simplest form of barrier method is the sheath, condom or French letter. This should be combined with spermicidal pessaries, cream, jelly or foam for greater safety. Used properly it has a failure rate of three pregnancies per 100 women per year. The advantages of this method are that the sheaths and spermicide can be bought in many shops and they are simple to use (read the instructions carefully if you are using them for the first time). The sheath has to be put on the erect penis and some couples find that stopping to put the sheath on interferes with the spontaneity of lovemaking. Some men find the sheath uncomfortable. An advantage of the sheath is that it protects both partners from infections and the cervix from sperm.

Diaphragm   The diaphragm or Dutch cap is another barrier method used together with spermicides. For this method to be comfortable and effective the vagina has to be measured by a gynaecologist so that the cap fits correctly within the vagina and over the cervix. Most women need a little practice before they can insert the cap, covered in spermicidal cream, easily and comfortably. When the diaphragm is in position it can be left there comfortably for some time. It is necessary to insert additional spermicide into the vagina if more than six hours have elapsed since the previous act of intercourse. This method protects the cervix from sperm. The failure rate is three pregnancies per 100 women per year. A similar device called the cervical cap, which is made from a mould of the woman's cervix and fits exactly, is being studied in several countries. There is little experience of this device being used by women with diabetes, but there is no reason why it should cause particular problems for them.

Intrauterine device (IUD)   The IUD or coil is inserted into the womb and by a combination of chemical and physical effects it prevents the fertilized egg from implanting there properly. Most gynaecologists prefer to give this only to women who have already had a pregnancy. The IUD has a failure rate of two pregnancies per hundred women per year. When it has been inserted by the doctor, it can be left in place and no other contraceptive measures need be taken.

There is a small risk of pelvic infection but there is no evidence that this is greater in diabetic women than in the general population. In rare cases, the infection may be so severe the women becomes permanently infertile. However, a few years ago, a more practical problem was noticed in diabetic users of the coil in Scotland. A large proportion became pregnant with the coil still inside the uterus. It was found that the coils removed from these women had different chemical deposits from those of non-diabetic women. These unusual chemicals had apparently made the coils ineffective. Newer coils are now available and appear to be as effective in women with diabetes as in non-diabetics.

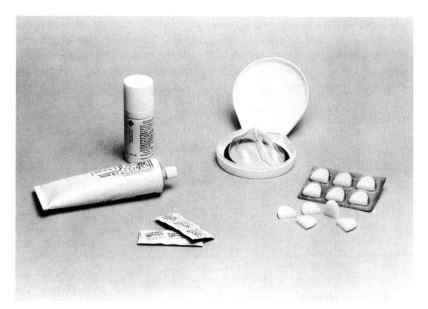

Recommended contraception: spermicidal jelly and foam, sheaths in foil packets, diaphragm or Dutch cap in box and spermicidal pessaries.

Pill The oral contraceptive pill, taken according to instructions, is the most effective way of preventing conception. The side-effects of the Pill are greater than those of other methods of contraception, but the failure rate is less than one pregnancy per hundred women per year.

However, diabetic women need to weigh the risks to their health of taking this hormone preparation. The Pill affects both glucose and fat metabolism. Both the oestrogen and the progestogen component can increase the body's intolerance to glucose. The increased insulin resistance may theoretically put the blood glucose level up in a treated diabetic. In practice this does not usually cause any problems because the dose of insulin can be adjusted. However, it may mean that a diet-treated diabetic finds it hard to control her glucose levels by diet alone. Oestrogens also increase the blood fats, triglycerides and cholesterol but progestogens do not. The Pill can cause high blood pressure (which may occur in people with diabetes anyway) and it is associated with blood clotting (thrombosis) problems, most commonly in the deep veins of the calf (called deep vein thrombosis). Atherosclerosis or hardening of the arteries may also develop or get worse and cause heart attacks or strokes. The risk of a heart attack or stroke through taking the Pill is probably greater in diabetics than in non-diabetics.

The risks of side-effects are greater in women over thirty-five years old, and much greater in women who smoke. These problems are related to the amounts of the two contraceptive hormones in the Pill. Nowadays, most Pills have a low oestrogen component and some contain progestogen only. Diabetic women, who decide with their doctor that they want to use the Pill, should certainly use a low-oestrogen one. Many doctors feel that the progestogen-only Pill is the most sensible choice.

Sterilization   A couple who have completed their family could consider vasectomy, or female sterilization by tying the Fallopian tubes, as alternatives. But do not take that decision lightly. You may want children later – possibly with another partner, and reversal of sterilization is not always easy.

Discussion   An unwanted pregnancy can be a disaster for all concerned, particularly if the woman has diabetes. Nowadays there is no excuse for unprotected intercourse, and this applies to men as well as women.

As soon as a diabetic girl has a relationship in which she thinks there is any possibility of sexual intercourse she should discuss contraception with her doctor. It is best to talk about contraception to whoever looks after your diabetes, but if this is difficult go to a Family Planning Clinic and make sure that you tell them you have diabetes. In an emergency, buy sheaths and spermicide.

I am often asked which is the best method of contraception for people with diabetes. My usual advice is that a barrier method (sheath or diaphragm with spermicide) properly used is best. However, if a couple find this method difficult or unacceptable they are less likely to use it properly than a couple who have themselves chosen a barrier method. Then, having discussed all the advantages and disadvantages, I suggest the progestogen-only Pill.

The decision about which of these methods to use should be shared between the couple and their doctor. Ultimately you should choose the one you feel that you and your partner will be able to use properly.

You should not forget your family in this discussion. Many young girls are afraid to talk about sex and contraception with their parents. It is always better to be open about things within the family, and most parents are more understanding than you imagine. After all, they have a sexual relationship and have probably experienced the same worries that you are having now.

Always bear the following points in mind:

- People with diabetes can enjoy sexual intercourse as much as anyone else, but do not forget that it uses energy.

- Impotence may trouble diabetic men in later years but it is commonly not due to diabetes and is often temporary. Do not bottle up your worries about this but discuss them with your doctor.
- If you are not planning a family, use contraception. Discuss the method of contraception most appropriate for you and your partner with your doctor before you have intercourse, not afterwards.

7 Having a family

People with diabetes can have happy, healthy families. Having diabetes does not prevent you from bearing normal children or from enjoying being a parent and giving your child a good start in life. However, like most health decisions in diabetes there are important factors to consider before making up your mind to have a baby.

Planning a family

There are several points which you need to consider as a diabetic man or woman planning to have a family:

1. Do both partners want to have a baby?
2. What risk is there of bringing a diabetic child into the world?
3. Will you be able to look after the child until he or she is old enough to look after him or herself?
4. If the woman has diabetes, is she fit enough to go through pregnancy and is her blood glucose normal?

The genetics of diabetes

Diabetes runs in families. This is true both for non-insulin-requiring and insulin-requiring diabetes. While there may be environmental factors affecting all members of a family, there is evidence that at least some of this family tendency to diabetes is inherited. It also seems that the type of diabetes breeds true; if you have insulin-dependent diabetes, other diabetics in the family will often also require insulin. Various research groups have studied the way in which diabetes is inherited. While it is possible to give an approximate idea of the risks of handing diabetes on to your family, it should be remembered that one population, for example, Canadian people, may behave differently from another, for example, British people, in terms of the pattern of inheritance. Also, the type of diabetes in your family may differ from that of another family. Unless every member is tested in a standard way, it is impossible to know how many people in a family have diabetes – and definitions of diabetes also vary.

Non-insulin-dependent diabetes This is also called Type II or maturity onset diabetes and it is likely that you will have had your children before you find out that you are diabetic. There is an uncommon form of young onset diabetes called Mason type (maturity onset diabetes of youth or MODY) which is dominantly inherited. That means that half your children will inherit it. For other forms of Type II diabetes, if one parent has it, 1 in 7 of the children eventually develop diabetes. If both parents have Type II diabetes, up to three quarters of their children will eventually become diabetic. If you have identical twins and one develops diabetes, the other will too. Non-insulin-dependent diabetes can develop at any age and it is possible that as many as 25 per cent of first-degree relatives (that is parents, brothers, sisters and children) of a non-insulin-requiring diabetic may become diabetic at some time. Because it may produce very few symptoms for many years, some of them may never know that they are diabetic.

Insulin-dependent diabetes The inheritance of insulin-dependent diabetes is easier to study because it usually produces severe symptoms and all family members with the condition are likely to know they have it. Some genetic markers are more likely to be found in people who are insulin-dependent diabetics than in those free from this condition. These are called the HLA antigens and are found on chromosome 6. People with either HLA-DR$_3$ or HLA-DR$_4$ are five times more likely to have insulin-dependent diabetes than those without these antigens. If you have both, the relative risk goes up to forty times. Many studies have looked at the brothers and sisters of insulin-dependent diabetics. Normally there is a one in four chance of two siblings sharing the same HLA genes. This increases to a one in two chance if both siblings have insulin-dependent diabetes. Further research has suggested that it is a gene close to the DR region called DQbeta which confers susceptibility to insulin-dependent diabetes. If one of the tiny components of the gene called aspartate is replaced by anything else in that particular position, the person may not be protected from developing diabetes if a trigger such as an infection appears later in life. Much work remains to be done and, as yet, these genetic markers are not specific enough to predict if someone is definitely going to become diabetic. If the mother has diabetes there is a one in a hundred chance that the child will develop diabetes. If the father has diabetes the risk of diabetes in his child increases to one in sixteen. If both parents have insulin-dependent diabetes the risk of their child developing diabetes may be as high as one in three, although older figures put it at one in twenty.

Age at diagnosis of diabetes   A Canadian study suggests that if you were aged under twenty years when your diabetes was diagnosed, your children are approximately twenty to forty times more likely to be diabetic than those of non-diabetic parents. If you were aged between twenty and forty when your diabetes was diagnosed, your children are approximately ten times more likely to be diabetic than those of non-diabetic parents. If you were over forty years old, your children are two or three times more likely to be diabetic. In a British study of newly diagnosed diabetics, 5 per cent of those under fifty years of age; 40 per cent of those between fifty and sixty-nine years and 30 per cent of those over seventy had a first-degree relative that is, a parent, sibling or child, who had diabetes.

Rare conditions   There are various very rare conditions in which diabetes plays a part and which are very strongly inherited. You will almost certainly know if you and other members of your family have a rare inherited condition associated with diabetes. In this case ask your doctor about the way it is inherited and the chances of your children having it.

Future generations   It is worth considering whether you are prepared to risk your child having diabetes and handing the condition on to future generations. The risk of passing on insulin-dependent diabetes may be less than that for non-insulin-requiring diabetes. However, a child with insulin-dependent diabetes may have to give himself injections for most of his or her life, whereas a non-insulin-dependent child may live most of his life free from diabetes. Obviously, we hope that medical advances will make diabetes easier to cope with in years to come.

Will you be able to look after your child?
Nowadays, most people with diabetes can look forward to a long and happy life. It is no longer unusual to meet people who have been on insulin for over fifty years and who have little trouble with their diabetes. However, some people with diabetes develop complications of the disease, and a very few are unfortunate enough to have severe complications such as heart disease or kidney disease at a time when they want to start a family. If this applies to you, you must face the fact that you may not be fit enough to help your children to grow up. This places an additional burden on your partner. If you and your partner are in this difficult situation, it is important to have some frank discussions with your doctor.

Am I fit enough to have a baby?

General health   No woman planning a family should smoke, drink a lot of alcohol or be too fat. Before you become pregnant, ask your doctor to check that you are immune to German measles (rubella) because it can cause severe damage to your baby if you catch it during the early months of pregnancy. If you are not immune your doctor can arrange for you to be vaccinated against rubella. As a person with diabetes you also need to know whether you have any complications of diabetes, such as high blood pressure or retinopathy, which may worsen during pregnancy; while if you have severe complications, you must consider the risk to your health if you become pregnant. Your doctor will advise you about this.

Blood glucose control   A vitally important factor is your blood glucose balance. For many years, doctors have known that good glucose control during pregnancy ensures that both mother and baby have the best possible chance of remaining healthy. But even with normal blood glucose levels from the first prenatal clinic visit onwards, more babies of diabetic mothers die than do those of non-diabetic mothers. The reason for this has become obvious over the past few years. Most women do not confirm that they are pregnant until the developing baby is several weeks old. The first eight weeks are critical in the development of the baby, because this is when most of the major body systems form. If the mother's blood glucose level is high at this time, this early development is upset and congenital abnormalities may occur. Some of these may be so severe that their baby does not survive. However, among women with diabetes whose blood glucose level is kept within normal limits from the moment of conception, the difference in their babies' survival and those of non-diabetic mothers virtually disappears.

Planned pregnancy   But how do I know when the moment of conception is? A diabetic mother-to-be must plan her baby and try to conceive only when her blood glucose levels are normal. Use contraception until you have your glucose balance right. Stopping barrier methods is less likely to cause a disturbance to your periods and your diabetic control than stopping the contraceptive Pill. For this reason, some doctors prefer that diabetic women planning to have a family use barrier methods of contraception. Some hospitals have pre-conception or pre-pregnancy clinics to help diabetic women plan their families. Ask if your hospital has one.

Pregnancy

Contact your doctor as soon as you suspect that you may be pregnant. Do not wait until you are sure. This means you should see him or her if your period has not appeared within a week of its expected day. Obviously it is more difficult to judge if your periods are irregular. Urine pregnancy tests have become more sensitive in recent years but it may be several weeks before you get a definite positive result. If you still have not had your period, keep checking the pregnancy tests.

A blood test can detect pregnancy much earlier than a urine test as tiny quantities of the hormone human chorionic gonadotrophin produced by the placenta are measured. This test is not available in all hospitals.

Normal glucose levels Both when you are planning your baby and when you are pregnant, you must have normal blood glucose levels. All your blood glucose tests must be between 4 and 6 mmol/l (72 and 108 mg/dl). Mild hypoglycaemia does not seem to harm the baby but severe hypoglycaemia may. Not only must you avoid high blood glucose levels, you must do so without going too low. No one pretends that this is easy. Having a baby is hard work for a diabetic mother. It is harder before pregnancy than when you are pregnant because the hormone changes which then occur act as a buffer to swings of glucose.

It is easier to measure such a small change in blood glucose levels with a meter, if you can borrow or buy one, as the colour changes on strips are very subtle. Pre-pregnant or pregnant diabetics should measure their blood glucose level four times a day before meals, with extra measurements if things do not seem right at other times, for example, after meals or during the night. Most clinics now also use the haemoglobin A_{1c} test (see Chapter 1) to check on the average blood glucose control during pregnancy.

Insulin You will almost certainly have to change to twice-daily insulin injections if you do not already need them, and may need more frequent injections of short-acting insulin during the day. It is usual in the UK to transfer diabetic women taking oral hypoglycaemic pills to insulin treatment before pregnancy, because of the potential risk of the pills damaging the developing baby. But do not panic if you find that you have become pregnant while taking oral hypoglycaemic drugs. Available reports and animal studies show no definite risk of teratogenicity, or imperfect development of the baby. If you have become pregnant while taking the pills, just change to insulin as soon as you know you are pregnant. You will probably be able to go back to your hypoglycaemic pills after delivery.

Some centres have used CSII pumps very successfully before and during pregnancy. Most rely on very close monitoring and frequent insulin injections.

Eat enough Your baby needs energy to grow. This means that you must increase your intake of food as your pregnancy progresses. Beware the dangerous habit of missing food because your blood glucose is a little high. It is easy for ketones to form during pregnancy and they are not good for developing babies. To keep ketones at bay you need insulin and carbohydrate.

Insulin requirements   Theoretically, if you have some insulin reserve of your own, your insulin need may fall during the first ten weeks of pregnancy. In practice, this is not often obvious and what most pregnant women with diabetes notice is a gradual increase in the insulin need, which is greater than you would expect from your increase in carbohydrate. This is because your body becomes increasingly insulin resistant owing to the hormonal changes of pregnancy. By the end of the ninth month you may be on twice the dose of insulin you were taking when your pregnancy started.

Delivery

In the old days, diabetic women were admitted to the hospital for months during their pregnancy, their babies were induced several weeks early and caesarian section was commonly performed. This was partly because poor glucose control led to very big babies. Nowadays, many obstetricians experienced in caring for diabetic women allow the pregnancy to come to term and vaginal delivery to take place.

Labour   When you go into labour, careful and continuous monitoring of you and the baby is started. A continuous glucose infusion is run into a vein with a continuous insulin infusion running at the same time. The rates of glucose and insulin infusion are adjusted according to your blood glucose levels. You will be given plenty of glucose because labour, as its name suggests, is hard work and if you do not have enough glucose, ketones will form which may harm the baby.

Do not be alarmed if a paediatrician or neonatologist is there when your baby is delivered. This is a precaution in case the baby has blood glucose problems while it is adjusting to living away from you. These are easily treated. Occasionally, babies of diabetic mothers have early breathing problems and these can be treated too. Sometimes, if there has been a period of poor glucose control during pregnancy, and occasionally even with perfectly controlled mothers, the baby is very large. If this happens you may need a caesarian section and the baby will probably be admitted to the special care baby unit for a few days. Your baby will be back with you as soon as the doctors have made sure that his or her glucose level is normal and the breathing is all right. The baby's weight will soon level off to match other babies of the same age.

Within a few hours of delivery your insulin requirements will drop dramatically. Therefore it is important that your glucose drip is not taken down until you are eating properly.

Today most diabetic women have healthy babies. If something goes wrong, do not blame yourself. Remember that a very small proportion of non-diabetic women also have babies with congenital problems, for no obvious reason. All you can do is try your best to keep yourself healthy during pregnancy and to keep your blood glucose normal; no one is perfect and no one can do more than her best.

Expert care   By now you will have realized that ensuring that women with diabetes keep well during pregnancy and labour and have healthy babies is a complex business. It is much better to travel a few extra miles to a hospital that has a special clinic for diabetic mothers than to go somewhere closer to home which rarely sees a pregnant woman with diabetes. Your diabetes adviser will know of local diabetic prenatal clinics, and he or she may even share one with an obstetric colleague.

If you have difficulties in finding expert care, your diabetic association (the American Diabetic Association — ADA — or the British Diabetic Association – BDA) may be able to tell where your nearest diabetic pre-natal clinic is. Home deliveries are out of the question for the diabetic mother-to-be.

After delivery

For all new mothers the weeks after delivery are ones of mixed feelings – the joy of your new baby; the sleepless nights; the worries about getting it right if this is your first child; the responsibilities of parenthood; and maybe a sense of anticlimax too. This can be especially acute in a diabetic mother. During pregnancy you have had very frequent clinic appointments and a lot of people have been deeply concerned about your general health and your diabetes. When you leave the hospital and your postnatal check-ups finish you may feel suddenly left alone. This is a time when husbands can be very supportive.

Breastfeeding

Diabetes is no deterrent to breastfeeding. You will continue to need plenty to eat while you are feeding your baby. Peggy, who comes to my clinic and has had three babies since becoming diabetic, thinks that she increases her diet by about 40 g carbohydrate a day while she is breastfeeding.

Your insulin requirements will have dropped after delivery and it may take a little while to get your insulin and diet right. It is important that you do not have hypoglycaemic attacks while you are holding your new baby in your arms and so it is better to run a little higher than you did during pregnancy to be sure that this does not happen. Aim for 6 or 7 mmol/l(108 or 126 mg/dl) rather than 4 mmol/l (72 mg/dl). When you stop breast-feeding, your dietary requirements may be reduced a little, although you may not notice any difference as you will have been weaning your baby gradually.

The diabetic mother

Being a mother and a housewife is as hard a job as any. Unlike most, it never stops. By the end of the day you may be worn out and still have to get up several times in the night to see to the children. During the time that you are looking after your family you may feel that your health takes second place to their needs.

Daisy is forty years old now and has brought up three children. Her husband works as a long-distance driver and is rarely at home. Daisy became diabetic when she was thirty-two years old. She was very over-weight and so was given a weight-reducing diabetic diet. Her weight fell a little, but her blood glucose levels rose and so she was started on glibenclamide pills. Over the years her glucose balance was never very good and when she was thirty-seven she was admitted to the hospital with abscesses and a very high blood glucose level. She was started on insulin.

Over the next few years Daisy had recurrent infections and several hospital admissions. Her weight went up and up and her average blood glucose level, measured in the clinic because she said she had no time to check it at home, was 17 mmol/l (306 mg/dl). She got more and more depressed. During this time she gradually told us what was going on at home. One of her daughters was mentally ill and in and out of psychiatric institutions. Her son was working but came home for all his meals. Her other daughter had started a feud with her grandmother, who also lived in the house, and the two of them were always bickering. The grandmother was not very well and needed a great deal of attention. Every Friday, Daisy had been going over to her sister's house to help with her cleaning, because her sister also had diabetes and couldn't cope; yet her sister had diet-treated diabetes and a fit husband.

It became apparent that Daisy was bearing all the family's burdens on her shoulders. She was neglecting herself and her diabetes completely, because she was so swamped by family chores. We suggested to Daisy that the time had come for her to think of herself and that she should ask her family to help her, not the other way around. Daisy was not too keen on this idea, but after her seventh hospital admission, she agreed to tackle her family. Since then she has lost forty pounds, she is measuring her own blood glucose levels, which are approximately 10 mmol/l (180 mg/dl) and sometimes lower, and the grandmother has gone to live with Daisy's diabetic sister, who now does her own cleaning – helped by her husband. Daisy's son is eating his lunch at work and her daughter is helping with the housework now that she has no one to argue with.

Obviously there are still problems, but at last Daisy's family have realized how ill she had become and have done something to help her.

Daisy's story is an extreme example, but I see many diabetic mothers in the clinic who are putting off coping with their diabetes 'until the family are grown up'. It may be too late then. Persistently high blood glucose levels may have done irreparable damage. Besides, you are not much use to your family if you make yourself ill. Looking after your diabetes does not take very much time when you get into a routine. The insulin and food pattern a housewife and mother needs is one for the person who has a variable work pattern (see Chapter 8 for how to adjust your insulin).

One of the difficulties for diabetic mothers is that they usually do the cooking and worry that the family will not like the diabetic diet. Most of the foods that are good for diabetics are those that any healthy family should eat. 'But my husband likes French fries, and sweet desserts'. Well, provide them occasionally. You do not have to eat them, although it is obviously a great temptation if you like them. One of my diabetic patients was a wonderful Viennese pastry chef and it used to break his heart not to be able to taste his creations.

The diabetic father

Most of this chapter has been written for women. As a diabetic father you may be the wage earner and so be particularly concerned about the effect your diabetes may have on your earning power. Provided you keep your diabetes under control, it should not interfere with your ability to do your job (see Chapter 8 for more about this aspect).

It is equally important for you as for your partner to consider the implications of having a family and you should consider carefully the points I discuss on pages 86–8. The physical implications are less crucial for the diabetic father. From the baby's point of view you need have no worries about your diabetic control at the time of conception. High glucose levels do not seem to upset the sperm.

The diabetic child

I have already discussed the question of inheriting diabetes. Parents often worry that their child may later become diabetic if one of them has diabetes. Even though they may have considered this before having a family and decided that the risk was small enough to continue, slight anxiety often remains.

The first point to make is that the sooner diabetes is treated the better. If you suspect that your child may have developed diabetes, do not just watch and worry. Check his or her urine or blood glucose and find out. If your fears are confirmed, go to your own doctor immediately.

But do not become obsessed with checking your child's urine for glucose. Unless both parents have diabetes, the odds are against your child being diabetic. If insulin-dependent diabetes does develop, it will be obvious very rapidly, because of the associated thirst, profuse urine and weight loss.

And if your child does develop diabetes? 'Doctor, I feel so guilty. It's all my fault. I've given it to her.' Yes, your genes did contribute, but other factors, many as yet unknown, triggered the diabetic process. You have also given your child her existence and a great deal more than the tiny fragment of genetic material which went towards her becoming diabetic. Your main job now is to help your child adjust to being a well-controlled diabetic as quickly as possible.

Always bear the following points in mind:

- Diabetic men and women can have happy, healthy children.
- It is important to plan your family.
- Consider the risks of passing on your diabetes to your children.
- Make sure that you are fit enough to go through pregnancy and look after your children afterwards.
- Plan to conceive at a time when your blood glucose is normal and tell your doctor as soon as you suspect that you may be pregnant. Keep your blood glucose normal throughout pregnancy but eat enough for your growing baby.
- Remember that insulin needs fall rapidly after delivery.
- Diabetes is no deterrent to breastfeeding.
- As your children grow up take care of yourself as well as your family.

8 Finding a job and working

Finding a job

I recently attended a diabetic meeting in an industrial Midlands town. In this area, and despite the high levels of unemployment, 95 per cent of people with diabetes who had attended a children's diabetic clinic found a job.

Beat the competition   Diabetes is not a barrier to getting most jobs. In the UK, people with diabetes are not allowed to enter the armed forces, the police force or, if insulin-treated, drive passenger-carrying or large goods vehicles. But the vast majority of trades and professions are open to people with diabetes with the right qualifications. Throughout the world jobs are becoming harder to get and it is therefore important for every young person, whether diabetic or not, to gain as many qualifications as he or she can before competing in the job market. This does not just mean academic qualifications, but generally being able to show that you are an interesting person. I must be realistic and say that if you have diabetes some potential employers may think twice before accepting you. This means that you must make sure that your qualifications for the job are as good as possible and preferably better than those of other competitors.

Applications   Virtually all jobs or opportunities for further training are gained through an application form, with or without a curriculum vitae, and an interview. Fill out the application form using a typewriter if you can. Otherwise print neatly. Ensure that the form is meticulously neat and that there are no mistakes. Type your curriculum vitae, having gone over it first with your careers guidance adviser or a senior colleague or friend. At this stage, unless specifically asked about health, do not advertise your diabetes. Some application forms ask for information on disabilities. Max, aged sixteen years, answered this question by saying, 'I have no disabilities, but I am a diabetic'. If asked, it is better to be honest about your diabetes than to conceal it.

When you are asked to go for an interview, look smart and neat – and conform. This is not the time to wear wild fashions unless, perhaps, you are applying to join a pop group. Do not allow your clothes or appearance to put off people in power (your future employer or head of college). When the subject of health comes up, or at an appropriate time during the interview, explain that you have diabetes but that it is well-controlled and does not interfere with your ability to work. You may have to explain exactly what diabetes is.

Medicals   Many organizations request a routine medical check on prospective members. Remember that the medical officer does not know you and your diabetes. Take your blood glucose diary to show your results (make certain that you know what they mean) and also to indicate that you are taking care of your diabetes. Make sure that you can reel off your precise dose and type of insulin and have your identity badge and emergency glucose to show. This may sound very naïve, but it is easy to get rattled in the heat of the moment, so write it all down too. A letter of support from your diabetic adviser may help.

Settling in to a new job

Learn your way around   Everyone is a little nervous about starting a new job. This applies whether it is your first job or your fifteenth. The first hurdle is to find your way around, and the initial landmarks are your work area, where you eat and the nearest lavatories. Within your work area find somewhere to keep some emergency snacks and canned drinks and also a quiet place in which to do your blood tests. The lavatory is not a good place to prick your finger because it is often dirty and cold.

Making friends   The next hurdle is getting to know all your new colleagues or workmates. As you get to know them, let them know about your diabetes. Do not make a great performance out of breaking the news, just let it come into the conversation naturally. When they know that you have diabetes, let them see that you do not mind discussing it. Then it will become an accepted part of working life and no longer strange or worrying for them. They should know what to do if you have a hypoglycaemic attack.

It is important that you feel relaxed enough to check your blood glucose in their company, if necessary, so that you can keep an eye on your diabetes at work. In every diabetic clinic, I meet people with diabetes whose blood glucose diaries contain gaps from nine in the morning to five in the evening. When I ask why, they reply, 'I can't check my blood glucose level at work because someone might see me.'

Some people with diabetes prefer to perform private urine tests during the working day and do blood tests at home. You can easily do urine tests by urinating on a reagent strip in the lavatory. This is a good way if your job is dirty, for example, in a machine shop or in building or garden work. On this point, if you have a job involving frequent contact with earth and mud, make sure that your tetanus injections are up to date.

A fixed work pattern

Many jobs have a fixed work pattern, by which I mean that you do similar things at similar times every day. These are fairly straightforward as far as diabetic balance is concerned. During the first few weeks, check your blood or urine glucose levels frequently and write the values down together with the activities which preceded or accompanied them. In this way, you will be able to work out how, if at all, you need to adjust your diabetic treatment to suit your job. If the job is very different from what you were doing before and you are finding it difficult to control your blood glucose, you may need to consider a different type of insulin or different timings of insulin injections. However, the problem can often be solved by adjusting the quantity and timing of your meals.

Joe is forty-seven years old and has worked on building sites for many years. He was recently promoted to the job of site foreman and now spends much of his working day sitting in the site office sorting out problems. He started putting on weight and his glucose levels went up. He was able to stop this trend by eating fewer sandwiches and snacks while at work and gradually cutting down on his insulin dose.

Shift work

If you have insulin-treated diabetes and have a choice of jobs, do not opt for shift work. Nevertheless, it is perfectly possible to keep good control of the blood glucose during shift work, so do not turn down a good job on that account. But it can take some hard thinking initially. The problem is not so much the shift itself as the times when life returns to normal at weekends: in other words, the variability of the work pattern. In many jobs involving shift work, it is possible to be given a regular shift pattern, for example, nights for a month, days for a month. This makes life a little easier.

Energy need When planning your therapy consider your energy need first. You should eat most before or during your times of greatest energy expenditure. If you are working a night shift, you need a good 'breakfast' in the evening and a substantial midnight meal.

When planning your insulin pattern it is helpful to think of the day as four separate periods: from getting up until the middle of the working day; the middle of the day until end of work; the end of work until bed-time; and

Chart 1 (top — early shift)

Date	Time	Urine Glucose	Urine Ketones	Blood Glucose	Insulin Dose	Remarks: — Hypos., Body Weight, Medications, Exercise, Colds, etc.
				AM 5 / 1700 PM	5 AM / 1700 pm	2 x Thyroxine 0.1mg Tablets Daily
Mon AUG 26				BM 7 / BM 7	12U VEL 6U VEL / 24U INS 14U INS	MON AUG 26 DAYS HOLIDAY SO WEEKENDS DOSE OF
Tue AUG 27				BM 7 \ BM 10	20U INS 6U VEL / ONLY 14U INS	INSULIN U100 AT 0600 AM INSULIN & BM AT
Wed AUG 28				BM 7 / BM 9	20U INS 6U VEL / ONLY 14U INS	1800 PM 26-AUG- 85
Thu AUG 29				BM 7 \ BM 4	20U INS 4U VEL / ONLY 14U INS	INSULIN AT 6.40 AM 1 SEPT
Fri AUG 30				BM 13 / BM 10	20U INS 6U VEL / ONLY 15U INS	
Sat AUG 31				BM 7 \ BM 13	24U INS 6U VEL / ONLY 14U INS	
Sun SEPT 1				BM 7 / BM 10	20+12U VEL 6U VEL 2 24U INS 14U INS	

Chart 2 (centre — late shift), U100

Date	Time	Urine Glucose	Urine Ketones	Blood Glucose	Insulin Dose U100	Remarks — Hypos., Body Weight, Medications, Exercise, Colds, etc
				AM 6 / PM 1800	AM 6 / PM 1800	2x Thyroxine 0.1mg Tablets daily
Mon 16 SEPT				BM 13 \ BM 10	8U VEL 14U INS / 20U INS ONLY	2 EXTRA UNITS OF VELOSULIN FOR HIGH BM
Tue 17 SEPT				BM 10 / BM 7	8U VEL 14U INS / 20U INS ONLY	SLIGHT LOSS OF CO-ORDINATION TOWARDS END OF SHIFT INDICATE
Wed 18 SEPT				BM BM BM 10 4 7	8U VEL 14U INS / 20U INS ONLY	POSSIBLE HYPO SO TOOK A MARS BAR FOR
Thu 19 SEPT				BM 7 / BM	8U VEL 14U INS 20U INS ONLY	SUGAR 19-9-85 INSULIN
Fri 20 SEPT				BM BM BM BM 7 4 7 10	8U VEL 14U INS 20U INS ONLY	LATE AT 0645AM BM 4 OBTAINED AT
Sat 21 SEPT				BM 7 / BM 13	8U VEL 6U VEL 24U INS 14U INS	DIABETIC CLINIC APPROX 11 00 AM 20/9/85
Sun 22 SEPT				BM 10 \ BM BM 13 10	12U VEL 6U VEL 24U INS 16U INS	21/9/85 2 EXTRA UNITS OF VELOSULIN FOR HIGH BM at 1800 PM

Chart 3 (bottom — holiday), U100

Date	Time	Urine Glucose	Urine Ketones	Blood Glucose	Insulin Dose U100	Remarks: — Hypos., Body Weight, Medications, Exercise, Colds, etc.
				6 / 1800 AM PM	6 / 1800 AM PM	2X 0.1mg THYROXINE TABLETS DAILY
Mon 23 SEPT				BM 7 \ BM 13	12U VEL 6U VEL / 24U INS 14U INS	EXTRA 2 UNITS FOR HIGH BM at 1800PM
Tue 24 SEPT				BM 13 / BM 9	12U VEL 4U VEL / 24U INS 14U INS	23-9-85 (VELOSULIN EXTRA 2 UNITS)
Wed 25 SEPT				BM 10 \ BM BM 4 2	12U VEL 4U VEL / 24U INS 14U INS	EXTRA SUGAR FOR LOW BM (MARSBARS)
Thu 26 SEPT				BM 7 / BM 7	BM 7 12U VEL 4U VEL 24U INS 14U INS	
Fri 27 SEPT				BM 10 \ BM 9	BM 7 12U VEL 6U VEL 24U INS 14U INS	2 EXTRA UNITS OF VELO-SULIN TO COPE WITH
Sat 28 SEPT				BM 13 / BM 13	12U VEL 4U VEL / 24U INS 14U INS	EXTRA FOOD AT PARTY 27/9/85
Sun 29 SEPT				BM 13 \ BM BM 7 4	12U VEL 4U VEL 24U INS 14U INS	

The records and blood glucose charts of a shift worker attending our clinic: *top*, early shift, *centre*, late shift, *bottom*, holiday.

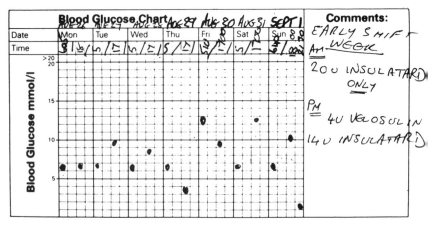

Blood Glucose Chart — AUG 29, AUG 30, AUG 31, SEPT 1

Comments:
EARLY SHIFT WEEK

AM 20 U INSULATARD ONLY

PM = 4 U VELOSULIN 14 U INSULATARD

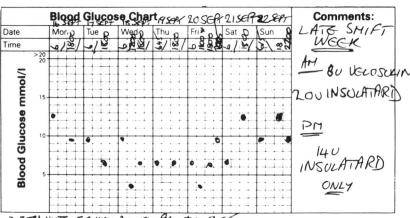

Blood Glucose Chart — 19 SEPT, 20 SEPT, 21 SEPT, 22 SEPT

Comments:
LATE SHIFT WEEK

AM 8 U VELOSULIN 20 U INSULATARD

PM 14 U INSULATARD ONLY

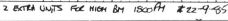

2 EXTRA UNITS FOR HIGH BM 1800 PM ≠ 22-9-85

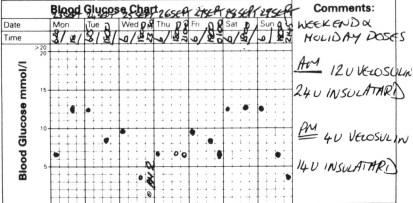

Blood Glucose Chart — 26 SEPT, 27 SEPT, 28 SEPT, 29 SEPT

Comments:
WEEKEND & HOLIDAY DOSES

AM 12 U VELOSULIN 24 U INSULATARD

PM 4 U VELOSULIN 14 U INSULATARD

sleeping. During this time you will have three meals, the first when you wake up, the second in the middle of the working day and the third at the end of the working day. You will also have snacks when necessary.

Insulin cover   Each of these periods of time needs insulin cover. Glucose balance on shift work is difficult to control on a once-daily insulin pattern. Either of the two most common patterns of insulin dosage can be adapted. Thus, rapid-acting and medium-acting insulin can be given in a larger dose to cover the larger meals and a smaller dose can be given for sleeping. The morning and evening quantities should be reversed when the waking and sleeping parts of the day are reversed. The other method is to use a very long-acting insulin as background and to add fast-acting insulin before breakfast and before your last big meal, adjusting the quantity as needed. On either regimen, extra doses of rapid-acting insulin can be added if necessary, before other meals or at times of changeover.

If you write down what you have done about meals and insulin and what effect it had on your blood glucose level you can use the successful regimen repeatedly as your shifts change during the year.

Pill treatment   People on pill treatment may also wonder what to do if they work shifts. If you are taking a once-daily dose of a long-acting oral hypoglycaemic (such as chlorpropamide) and you take it in the morning every day regardless of when you are sleeping or working, you may find your blood glucose level dropping much too low during a sleeping day and rising too high during a working night. If you take it before 'breakfast', whether this is in the evening or morning, you may take two pills within twenty-four hours on one of your changeover days. Again, your blood glucose level may drop too low. This may not happen if you are on a very small dose of chlorpropamide, but you should keep a careful eye on your blood glucose level whatever dose you are on. It may be easier to manage shift work with short-acting pills such as tolbutamide or glipizide. These should be taken at meal times, whether during the day or at night. In practice, the simplest solution seems to be small doses of a short-acting hypoglycaemic pill at each meal time.

Variable work pattern
Some jobs, for example medicine, sales work or journalism, have an unpredictable work pattern. It is often impossible to know how much energy you will need from one day to the next and, in some jobs, even where you will be. If you are moving from a fixed routine job to a variable one, you may be startled by the disruption this causes in your glucose balance. In some cases, people with previously well-balanced diabetes find they have high glucose levels one hour and are hypoglycaemic the next.

There are various ways of coping with this and to some extent the method you choose is influenced by your diabetic adviser. Generally, it is easier to take a long or extremely long-acting insulin (for example, Ultratard) to provide some background insulin throughout the day and night and to add small, frequent amounts of rapid-acting insulin to this as required. The same principle applies to food. Eat a steady amount of high fibre food during the day to provide a relatively constant carbohydrate input and boost this by more rapidly absorbed carbohydrate to cover periods of exertion. Frequent blood glucose tests are needed, particularly just before you begin an activity during which hypoglycaemia would be dangerous, such as driving.

Controlling fluctuating glucose levels   The first rule is not to keep altering your insulin dose. It takes several days for the effect of a change in a long-acting insulin dose to become apparent. Furthermore, if you change two types of insulin at once it may be hard to judge the effect, especially if you are also altering your food intake. To start with, make sure that you do not go hypoglycaemic, so run a little on the high side. Then take each part of the day in turn and bring the blood glucose levels down towards normal by adjusting your food intake. Try adjusting your insulin only when food adjustments have failed. This process may take two or three weeks so a little patience is needed. If things start going badly awry do not struggle on but ask for help. It may be that you would be better on another insulin regimen.

Pills or diet alone
Much of what has been said above also applies to people on oral hypoglycaemic treatment. In general, people treated with pills or diet alone have less dramatic swings in blood glucose level than those taking insulin. Nevertheless, good glucose balance is as important. The need to adjust energy input to balance output is the same whatever form of treatment you are using. The dose or the timing of pills may need to be altered, for example, as I described for shift work. Hypoglycaemia is less common among people on pills and may catch you unawares when a heavier workload precipitates your first attack.

The businessman or woman

In the tough world of business it is important that your diabetes does not dull your competitive edge. Indeed, in some business deals, a badly timed hypoglycaemic attack could lose millions! It is also important that controlling your diabetes does not interfere with your work. Therefore you must strike a balance between the time and effort needed to maintain good glucose control and the interference to your lifestyle that these efforts can cause; not forgetting the immediate and longterm damage that poor glucose control can cause.

Gadgets   If you are well off financially, you may be able to afford the aids that can make diabetic life easier and more comfortable. These include blood glucose measuring meters or biosensors. But money does not buy personal expertise, and there have been problems with people who have bought themselves CSII pumps without adequate back-up and failed to learn how to use them properly.

Meetings   The life of the typical businessman includes frequent meetings, large dinners with alcohol, long-distance travel and much stress. While many businessmen do not live like this all the time, most will encounter some of these facets at one time or other.

Meetings rarely begin or finish on time. They are periods of physical inactivity, when you are usually trapped in a smoke-filled room. Yet it is important not to fall asleep or to leave the room as your opponents will use the opportunity to their advantage, while your friends will promptly volunteer you for some thankless task. In your briefcase you should include something to eat that is unobtrusive, your emergency glucose, your blood testing kit and your insulin (this is where a preloaded syringe, Novopen, BD-Lilly pen or Pur-in pen is helpful – see Chapter 2). If you have enough to eat and your insulin, you can sit out any meeting that is overrunning without worrying about your diabetes.

Obviously it is preferable not to have to check your blood glucose level or to give insulin during a meeting, but both can be done surreptitiously if essential, and if you are among friends aware of your diabetes it should not matter. I once saw a very eminent physician with diabetes give an injection of insulin while sitting on a platform chairing a meeting of several hundred people. I doubt if many of those present noticed him slip his preloaded syringe out of his pocket and inject the insulin because it was done in seconds. The easiest site is the abdomen. Just undo the lower buttons on your shirt and inject the insulin. Injecting through tights or trousers is possible but not very hygienic, and is not to be recommended.

As a general principle, it is better to inject insulin quickly in public than to retreat into a lavatory and acquire an infected injection site. This also removes the unfortunate suspicion that the man slipping quietly into the lavatory with a syringe is a junkie.

Meals   Business dinners are traditionally high in sugar, fat and alcohol. However, any reasonable restaurant should be able to offer alternatives that fit in with a diabetic diet. A grilled steak with potatoes and salad followed by fresh fruit and bread and cheese is one possibility available in most cities. If in doubt as to the contents of a tempting dish, ask the waiter or the chef.

Alcohol

People with diabetes do not have to become teetotal, but alcohol can upset glucose balance in several ways. First, it is a source of calories and must be considered as part of the day's calorie input. Second, and more important, it reduces the amount of glucose released into the circulation by the liver. This means that there is a risk of hypoglycaemia after drinking alcohol. After a heavy night's drinking, alcohol is likely to be circulating in the blood the next morning. In practical terms, this means that a person with diabetes, particularly if insulin-treated, who has some alcohol in the evening may become hypoglycaemic on the way home, that night or the next morning. Always have something to eat with an alcoholic drink.

Tony is forty-two years old, on twice-daily insulin injections and works in a sports shop. He drank one and a half pints of 'sugar-free' beer after work. On his way home he was stopped by the police while driving erratically and was promptly treated as a drunk driver because his breath smelled of alcohol and he was confused and aggressive. A breath test was negative but he was taken to the police station because of his behaviour. Unfortunately, he did not bother to carry a diabetic card and no one realized that he was diabetic.

Later that night Tony was found unconscious in the cells. When he was transferred to the hospital, a blood check revealed that his glucose was 1 mmol/l (18 mg/dl). He was revived with an intravenous glucose injection.

Tony could not believe that as little as one and a half pints of beer could have had such a severe effect on his glucose level. One of the things he did not know was that 'sugar-free' beer has less carbohydrate in it because the brewing process is taken further. The excess carbohydrate is converted into more alcohol. Also, when someone has had nothing to eat, even a small amount of alcohol can induce hypoglycaemia.

Alcohol flushing Alcohol may produce another problem for people on pill treatment. About 60 per cent of those on chlorpropamide develop facial flushing within half an hour of drinking alcohol. For a few people this reaction can be very distressing with a feeling of severe burning in the face, and sometimes all over the body, nausea, wheezing and faintness. Whether you get this alcohol flushing depends to some extent on the dose of chlorpropamide you are taking and when you last took it. It is less likely to

104

Approximate calorie and carbohydrate values for some alcoholic drinks

Drink	Kilocalories	Available carbohydrate grammes
Beer	30 kcal/100 ml 170 kcal/pint	2–3 g/100 ml 11–17 g/pint
Stout	40 kcal/100 ml 230 kcal/pint	2–4 g/100 ml 17–23 g/pint
Cider	40–100 kcal/100 ml 230–570 kcal/pint	3–7 g/100 ml 17–40 g/pint
Port	160 kcal/100 ml 80 kcal/50 ml glass	12 g/100 ml 6 g/50 ml glass
Sherry Dry – sweet	110–140 kcal/100 ml 55–70 kcal/50 ml glass	1–7 g/100 ml 1–4 g/50 ml glass
White wines Champagne	70 kcal/100 ml 80 kcal/113 ml glass	1 g/100 ml 2 g/113 ml glass
Dry – sweet	70–90 kcal/100 ml 80–100 kcal/113 ml glass	3–6 g/100 ml 3–7 g/113 ml glass
Red wines	70 kcal/100 ml 80 kcal/113 ml glass	<1 g/100 ml <1 g/113 ml glass
Spirits 70% proof	220 kcal/100 ml 50 kcal/24 ml glass	trace trace

One pint (20 fl oz) = 568 ml
1000 ml = 1l = 1.76 pints
One US pint (16 fl oz) = 454 ml

happen with other sulphonylurea drugs, such as glibenclamide, and the simple solution if you have this problem is to change your pills. About 6 per cent of the population are born with the tendency to flush with alcohol. So, if you are a born alcohol flusher, you will either have to put up with it or stop drinking.

Stress
Stress is by no means limited to business people. There is little scientific evidence that stress causes diabetes. However, many people with diabetes find that their blood glucose level goes up at times of stress.

Martin, forty-eight years old, works in a car factory. He is also a union shop steward. Normally, his diabetes is well-controlled, but one afternoon he came into clinic with a glucose level of 20 mmol/l (360 mg/dl). He had just had a furious argument with his fellow shop stewards who wanted to call the men out on strike over an issue with which he disagreed. He told me later that it took two days for his glucose levels to come down after this incident.

Finding a job and working

- Diabetes is not a barrier to getting most jobs.
- Make sure that your qualifications are as good as or better than any non-diabetic competitor.
- When applying for jobs be honest.
- Tell your friends and colleagues about your diabetes. There is no need to be ashamed or embarrassed about it.
- Consider your work pattern when organizing your diet and diabetes treatment. A little forward planning can make life easier. Ensure that you arrange for a new family doctor and diabetes adviser if you leave home.

9 Exercise

Exercise is good for anyone with diabetes. It helps keep your weight down, increases your sensitivity to insulin, tones your muscles, encourages your circulation, helps your heart and makes you feel good. You can 'fine tune' your blood glucose by balancing food, treatment and exercise. Regular sensible exercise is an excellent means of relaxation and often a source of good companionship.

What happens when you exercise
Glucose   The main source of energy for exercising muscles is glucose. It is constantly circulating in the blood stream ready to be taken up by the cells. Approximately half of this glucose is converted into energy immediately, one-fifth is stored as glycogen in the liver and a quarter is stored as glycogen in the muscles. Glucose cannot enter any cells without insulin. Insulin is also essential for glucose to be converted into glycogen stores in the muscles. As the muscles work, the glycogen is broken down to provide glucose for energy. As the muscle glycogen is used up, more glucose is taken from the blood stream to provide more energy. The liver releases glucose from its glycogen stores to meet the increased energy need. At the same time, fat and protein are also used to provide energy. If insulin is not available, or if the liver glycogen stores are exhausted, the exercising muscle has to rely entirely on fat and protein breakdown for energy once it has used up all its glycogen stores (see ketoacidosis, page 49). Excess insulin stops the release of glucose from the liver stores.

Insulin sensitivity   As exercise continues, the body, and the muscles in particular, become more sensitive to the action of insulin. This means that a given dose of insulin helps more glucose to be used by the body. In practical terms, it means that someone with diabetes who starts a regular exercise training programme needs fewer oral hypoglycaemic pills or less insulin a day to control his or her blood glucose, even if the body weight stays the

Exercise, food and insulin

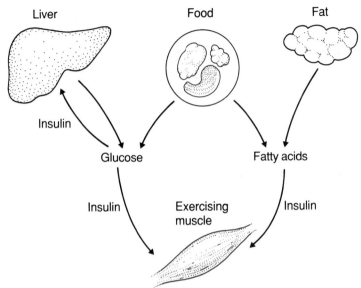

Liver

Food

Fat

Insulin

Glucose

Fatty acids

Insulin

Exercising muscle

Insulin

	At rest	Brief exercise	Longer exercise
Food	Glucose and fat absorbed into the blood	Glucose and fat absorbed into the blood	Less glucose and fat absorbed as some blood diverted to muscle
Insulin normal	Released from the pancreas according to blood glucose	Less insulin released from pancreas as glucose falls	
diabetic	Released from the injection site	More released from injection site as circulation to muscles and skin increases	
Liver	Stores glucose as glycogen*	Starts to release glucose^	Releases a lot of glucose^
Fat	Stores fatty acids*	Starts to release fatty acids^	Releases a lot of fatty acids^
Muscle	Stores glucose as glycogen*	Converts glycogen to glucose for energy*	Takes up glucose and fatty acids and uses them for energy*

* Needs insulin
^ Blocked by insulin

same. This increase in insulin sensitivity happens both to diabetics and non-diabetics. It appears rapidly and disappears equally rapidly when you stop exercising regularly.

Reorganization of body glucose stores After each bout of exercise the body reorganizes its glucose stores. The muscles start to build up glycogen again. The waste products of exercise are cleared from the blood stream. Obviously, hypoglycaemia can occur during exercise because glucose is used to produce energy. However, it can also occur during reorganization of glucose stores. This sort of hypoglycaemic attack can take place several hours after you have finished exercising. It may happen at night, even after you have eaten a large meal. You may find you need extra carbohydrate before, during and after strenuous exercise.

These changes in your body's metabolism mean that if you start a regular exercise programme you will need to eat more (unless you are trying to lose weight) and take less insulin or fewer oral hypoglycaemic pills. The amount by which the food should be increased and insulin decreased varies for each person and each activity. If you continue a regular exercise pattern for months, your diet and insulin dose will stabilize. You will need to protect yourself against hypoglycaemic attacks during and after exercise.

Can exercise be dangerous for diabetics?
Yes, under some circumstances: You should not exercise hard when you are showing moderate or heavy ketones in the urine. You should not exercise when you are hypoglycaemic, but wait until you have corrected this. While exercising keep your heart rate within the training zone for your age.

Your age in years	Your heart rate in beats per minute	
	60% maximum	85% maximum
20	120	187
30	114	161
40	108	153
50	102	144
60	96	136
70	90	127

Training zone for exercise

The level of exercise you choose is also important. If you are young and relatively fit, a few hours' very energetic exercise will do little damage. If you are over forty, overweight, unfit and suffer from angina, a game of squash could kill you. Do not rush in, but take it gradually. Exercise regularly (three times a week is often recommended) and gradually increase the length and amount you do at each session. Another book in this series, *The Diabetics' Get Fit Book* by Jacki Winter, will help you choose the right exercise programme.

Types of exercise

Sprinting

This is an example of the 'quick burst' type of exercise. Sprinting is not the type of exercise for the unfit older amateur to choose. You need a lot of energy in a very short time. This can be provided beforehand by rapidly absorbed carbohydrate, such as a glucose drink. More rapidly absorbed and some slowly absorbed carbohydrate will be needed afterwards. A small insulin reduction may be necessary.

Marathon running

This is an example of endurance exercise. A marathon runner builds up to a distance of many miles by gradually increasing training runs over a long period of time.

If you take up this type of running you need to consider how far you usually run and at what time of day, and reduce your insulin accordingly. You will need slowly absorbed carbohydrate food and some instant energy before you start. The instant energy, for example in the form of slightly salted glucose drinks, will need to be repeated at frequent intervals along the track, probably every one or two miles, to top up your energy and fluid supplies. After the race you will have to take more rapidly absorbed and plenty of slowly absorbed carbohydrate to counteract late falls in glucose.

Water sports

There is no reason why people with diabetes should not go swimming. Swimming exercises the whole body. If you go to a pool regularly you can increase the number of lengths or widths that you swim gradually, so it is a good exercise for the older diabetic.

The risk is that the exercise will make you hypoglycaemic and that you will become unconscious and drown, but this is preventable. First, never swim alone and do not go out of your depth if the person with you is not capable of rescuing you from deeper water (in any case, it is better to choose a companion who can swim). Second, immediately before entering the water, you must ensure that you have eaten enough to fuel your swim, but not overfilled your stomach. Eat a high fibre meal about one to two hours before swimming and have some rapidly absorbed carbohydrate, such as glucose, just before you enter the water. Carry glucose with you in the

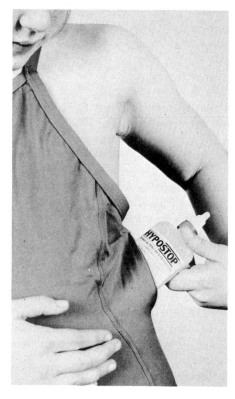

Glucose gel can be safely carried in a swimming costume.

water; hard-boiled candies can be knotted into a plastic bag pinned to your bathing suit. Hypostop glucose gel comes in a small polythene bottle which is water-resistant and can be carried in a pocket in your bathing suit. If you are in the water for a long time, have a snack halfway through.

People with diabetes are prone to cramp, and this may be reduced by drinking bitter lemon or tonic, both of which contain quinine. The possibility of cramp is another reason why you should not swim alone. Do not allow yourself to get chilled; cold and hypoglycaemia do not mix (see page 144).

If you have not been swimming before, or not recently, check your blood glucose level before and after swimming to see what effect this exercise has had on you.

Swimming in the sea is more hazardous. It can be done by diabetics, but you must take all the precautions described above and remember the added dangers. Never go far from land out of your depth, especially where there are big waves or unknown currents.

Winter sports

Skiing Skiing courses are now offered to people with diabetes in several countries including Britain, the USA and Norway. Like any other form of exercise it is important to start gradually and learn how the activity affects you and your diabetes. This may be difficult if you have only a week on the slopes in which to learn to ski and to cope with the weather, new food and everything else. If you can, practise on a dry ski slope first so that you have learned the basic moves before you leave home.

Good, well-fitting equipment is very important. It is vital that your boots are comfortable, because any soreness may spoil your holiday and rubs and blisters may take a long time to heal. Take your time choosing your foot-wear and do not be hurried into a bad decision. Remember that you usually get what you pay for; it may be worth paying a little more for comfort. Cold is one hazard, especially if you have poor circulation. I even saw two diabetics with frostbite in Oxford one winter. So wear proper ski gloves and make sure your feet are kept warm, particularly if you are doing a lot of standing around in very cold conditions. Your ski equipment shop will advise you on the best type of socks to wear inside your boots.

Another problem is glare from the sun and snow. Many skiers suffer from sunburnt faces so do not forget to put sunscreen on your face, and wear a pair of protective goggles to save you from snow blindness.

Although the beginners' slopes may be near the hotel, as you progress you will be going farther and farther up the mountain and you may spend the whole day away from base. It is important that you have enough food not only to last for expected meals and snacks but to cope with unexpected delays. Your food should include plenty of rapidly absorbed glucose. The bum bag or ski bag described in Chapter 10 comes in handy here and will not impede your skiing. Take your insulin and syringes or pen with you too, but do not allow the insulin to freeze. For skiing well away from base the precautions prescribed in the mountain expeditions section of Chapter 10 apply.

If you have an accident it is vital that you do not become hypoglycaemic and cold. You should eat some glucose if you feel hypoglycaemic and have to wait in the snow to be rescued, even if you are going to need an anaesthetic to set a broken leg. When the doctor arrives, tell him what you have eaten, when and why.

What about the après ski? You have earned it and need to replace all the calories and carbohydrate the skiing has used up. Take alcohol in moderation though, because it may prevent your body from reorganizing its glucose stores after all your exercise. If you spend the evenings at a disco, remember to take an extra snack and insulin with you (see Chapter 5).

Winter mountain walking All the comments about mountain expeditions in Chapter 10 apply here. In winter conditions all mountains are dangerous and require special skill and expertise. The pretty view of the snow-capped mountains reflected in the lake in the chocolate box picture conceals glass-slippery ice, snow-covered holes and gullies, treacherous snow slopes and avalanches, and was produced by a blizzard which may well recur. This also applies a few yards from the ski slopes, so beware the temptation to take a stroll off the beaten track. Take local advice about walking. If it is snowy enough to ski you will almost certainly need proper winter walking equipment with ice axes and crampons, and these cannot be used unless you have been trained to handle them properly.

Remember that walking in snow warmed by the sun is extremely hard work and uses enormous amounts of energy. If you are setting off on foot, get up very early so as to complete most of your walk (especially the uphill bit) before the snow has softened. Having said all this, I think the mountains are beautiful in winter and well worth exploring. My comments apply to people with and without diabetes and non-diabetics alike. Those with diabetes can derive as much enjoyment from winter walking as anyone else.

Tennis and squash
Tennis and squash are good sports to take up if you travel because many cities have squash and tennis courts and the equipment is not bulky to carry. They present no particular problems if you have diabetes. Squash has increasingly become a game for professional people and business-men, and it is being taken up by more mature people. It is a demanding and exciting game and requires a high level of fitness. As with all other sports, start training gradually and do not place sudden and unexpected demands on your body. Practise on your own to start with and build up to full matches. Squash is not an appropriate game for people who have heart trouble.

Sports courses or vacations
One sort of course involving one or two weeks of concentrated exercise is described in Chapter 10. Many vacations, however, include sporting activities. If you go on one of these to learn sailing or improve your tennis, for example, you will need to reduce your insulin or pills and increase your food intake during the relatively short periods of intensified exercise. The effect of greater insulin sensitivity will become increasingly obvious.

Team sports
There are people with insulin-treated diabetes in many well-known sports teams, for example, in football, swimming and hockey. They have a duty not only to themselves to perform well but also to their team, county or country. At this level of sport, you will be training regularly and exercise will be part of your daily routine. Each diabetic

player must work out for himself how much to eat before a match and what to eat at half-time. Important matches may also cause you stress, which may increase or decrease your insulin need. Added to this is the effect of travel before and after the match (see Chapter 8). Your diabetic preparations should be included in your pre-match ritual.

Exercises for people with special problems

Heart disease
People with diabetes are at greater risk of heart trouble than non-diabetics (see Chapter 4). If you have angina or have had a heart attack, do not assume that you will never be able to exercise again and that you must lead the life of an invalid. The right sort of exercise will help your heart. The first thing to do is to find out from your doctor exactly what has happened to your heart. Then ask what sort of exercise you can do safely.

Heart attack   If you have had a heart attack you will probably be told to rest in bed for the first few days, then be allowed to sit out of bed, and within a couple of weeks be walking increasing distances on flat surfaces, in the hospital or at home. After this the usual advice is to do a little more each day, on flat surfaces to start with, then up stairs and inclines, gradually increasing the speed and length of your walks.

Some cardiologists ask people who have had a heart attack to do a gentle exercise test on a treadmill within a few weeks of the attack to see how the heart behaves under supervised exercise and to assess the need for further treatment. Increasingly, hospitals are running training sessions in the gymnasium for people who have recovered from an attack.

Angina is nearly always brought on by exertion and this may stop you from exercising at all. Nowadays, with a wide range of medication to choose from and the option, where appropriate, of coronary artery bypass surgery, people with angina need not spend the whole time resting. In fact, this is definitely not good for them. Get yourself thoroughly tested by your doctor or a cardiologist, take your recommended treatment and then ask about gently increasing the amount you do each day. Your doctor will be able to show you how to count your pulse and what the maximum rate should be when you exercise. It may be possible to get back to normal with the right treatment.

One class of drugs used to treat angina, the beta-blockers (remember the -olol drugs mentioned on page 61) sometimes make your muscles feel very tired. This is especially likely with non-selective beta-blockers, so a change to a selective one may help. Other drugs, the nitrates, make your blood vessels dilate. Nitrates come in many forms, including pills that can be taken under the tongue, or skin patches. If you inject your insulin into your arm and stick your nitrate skin patch on that arm you may find that your insulin is absorbed very rapidly. It would then obviously be better to alter the site where you put the patch.

Legs

Atherosclerosis of the large blood vessels of the legs may cause pain in your calves (and sometimes thighs or buttocks) when you walk. This is called intermittent claudication (see Chapter 4). I cannot ever remember seeing someone with intermittent claudication who did not smoke. As I said before, people with diabetes do not smoke.

If your legs hurt, you do not want to walk, but with this condition it is important that you do. While you keep exercising the legs, collateral vessels will open up to bypass the blocked and narrowed ones and improve the circulation. Walking is one of the best exercises to help intermittent claudication. Set yourself a target distance to walk and add a few yards to it every day. You will find that you have to stop less and less frequently to let your legs recover.

Exercises at home can help too. Hold on to the back of a firm chair and raise yourself up and down on your toes several times. Sit down and lift your legs up and down off the floor. Then lift them straight up in front of you and make circles with your toes, rotating your feet at the ankles. Go to the bottom of the stairs or find a firm stool to put near your chair and do a few step ups (see the photographs opposite). Start gently at first and then do more of each exercise and move more quickly.

Eyes

If you have proliferative retinopathy you should not exercise until your opthalmologist says you can. Vigorous exercise could cause new vessels to bleed.

Exercise for the not-so-young

Whatever your age, you can benefit from a little exercise. For mature people not used to sport, walking is good exercise, with the benefits of fresh air and a changing view to keep you from getting bored. Try a short walk every day. Early morning stretching and flexing of your arms and legs, like a cat when it wakes up, helps to keep you supple. There are many exercise programmes that give you specific exercises to follow. The general rule is to do it gradually and not to do anything that hurts.

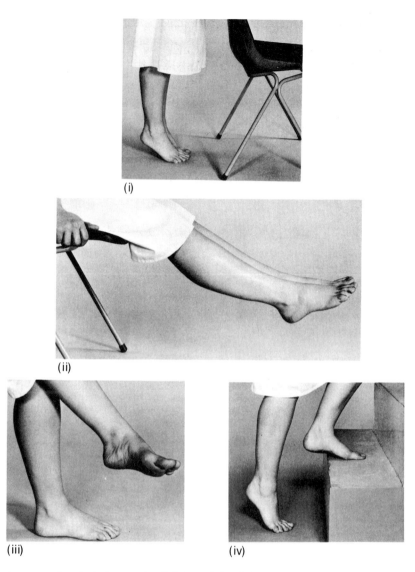

(i)

(ii)

(iii)

(iv)

Leg exercises to help muscles, joints and circulation: (i) supporting yourself with a chair back, raise yourself gently up and down on your toes (ii) sitting on the chair with your legs outstretched, raise and lower them slowly (iii) cross one leg over the other and describe circles with your toes; practise in both directions and with both feet (iv) practise step ups alternately, giving a good stretch to the muscles of both legs. Begin with a few repetitions of each exercise and build up gradually.

Always bear the following points in mind:

- Exercise is good for people with diabetes. It increases your glucose utilization and your insulin sensitivity.
- Eat more and take fewer pills or less insulin when you exercise.
- Take the type of exercise you enjoy and that you can manage safely. Do not pretend to yourself that you are fit when you are not. Grade your exercise.
- If you have complications of diabetes, ask your doctor about exercise. It may help your condition.
- You are never too old to exercise; and if you exercise regularly it will make you feel good and keep you fit.

10 Diabetes Outward Bound

In 1981, the British Diabetic Association (BDA) and the Outward Bound (OB) Trust together established the first Outward Bound course for insulin-treated diabetic teenagers. At that time, some people said it was impossible for diabetics to complete such an energetic course and that activities such as climbing and abseiling were too dangerous for anyone taking insulin. Paul, aged sixteen years, who came on the eighth BDA/OB mountain course, told me that he had been banned from his canoeing club when he became diabetic. Yes, the eighth course. The first group of sixteen diabetics proved that they were as capable of completing an OB course as any group of non-diabetic teenagers. Since 1981, there have been over twenty-five BDA/OB courses for people with diabetes ranging in age from fourteen to sixty-four years, and on all forms of treatment. In 1991 we had our ten year reunion.

This chapter describes the way the students on these courses learn how to adapt their diabetic management to a very strenuous one or two weeks. The lessons learned illustrate some ways of coping with situations in which there is a variable and frequent energy need, varying meal times and also potential danger.

Behind the scenes

Most of the participants on these courses do not realize that, long before they arrive, a great deal of planning has gone on behind the scenes. Before the first course a dietitian and I went up to the OB centre at Eskdale in the Lake District to discuss the activities with the course director. It all sounded rather alarming to us, but right from the beginning I had decided that the BDA group was going to try all the activities of an ordinary course. If we were going to do it, we were going to do it properly. I copied down a list of the planned activities and exactly what they entailed, and noted the daily timetable. Then I took it home and thought very hard.

The aim was for all participants to enjoy and complete the course successfully without their diabetes getting in their way, but without losing control of their blood glucose. How could I ensure that the participants would be as safe as humanly possible? What was the worst that could happen? It all seemed to boil down to one major hazard – hypoglycaemia. We needed to protect the participants from the risk of going hypoglycaemic and falling off something, falling into water, getting confused, getting lost or getting injured. If someone with diabetes is exercising hard, he or she is more likely to become hypoglycaemic. Furthermore, we would be spending our time in a mountainous area, several hours from the nearest telephone and at least twenty miles (thirty-two kilometres) from the nearest hospital.

The first step was to ensure that the applicants for the course were in reasonable control of their diabetes. An OB course is not the place to try to sort out someone with grossly uncontrolled diabetes. I later learned that application forms rarely give you as much information as you need on the applicant's degree of control, and that some of the participants may be in a dreadful muddle with themselves and their diabetes.

Everyone with diabetes is different and everyone responds individually to treatment and different situations. Warning signs of hypoglycaemic attacks are different. It was therefore very important that all the helpers on the BDA and OB teams got to know all the students as soon as possible. I had a talk with every participant on arrival, and discussed his or her diabetes, general health and any worries about the course.

Blood glucose levels   In order to prevent hypoglycaemic attacks we needed to know what was happening to every participant's blood glucose level. We taught all the participants who were not already checking their blood glucose how to do so and what the results meant. I decided that to be safe I would ask all the participants to run their blood glucose levels higher than is normally acceptable. We aimed for 10 mmol/l (180 mg/dl) rather than 4 mmol/l (72 mg/dl) to allow for rapid falls in glucose during exercise.

Fuel for exercise   We increased everyone's diet by doubling the carbohydrate in all snacks right from the beginning, and then gradually increasing the main meals throughout the course. I was astonished by the amount the students needed to eat, and so were they. Some of them doubled their total daily carbohydrate intake and still had blood glucose levels of 7–10 mmol/l (126–180 mg/dl). We used normally forbidden foods, such as chocolate and sweet biscuits or cookies, to provide rapidly absorbed energy during exercise, and glucose tablets immediately before anything potentially dangerous, such as climbing.

Insulin One of our problems was that no one knew by how much the insulin dose needed to be reduced on such a constantly energetic course. On the first course, I suggested reducing the insulin by a few units on the first day, and if the blood glucose levels were under 7 mmol/l (126 mg/dl) or hypoglycaemic attacks occurred, I reduced it further. The participants and I were all surprised by the final insulin reductions. The body very rapidly becomes sensitized to insulin with regular strenuous exercise.

Safety We did all we could to prevent attacks occurring. But what about the unexpected severe one that might cause unconsciousness? Safety standards are high at all OB centres. Safety ropes are used for climbing and life-jackets on the water. Activities are supervised by highly trained and experienced instructors. We used one simple rule to assess all activities – if the student suddenly becomes unconscious will he still be safe? We found that existing safety standards at the OB centres already covered this. We decided that students should not do solo activities and we ensured that all instructors and students were taught how to deal with a hypoglycaemic attack, even a severe one. All activities were accompanied by OB instructors and BDA staff, if necessary linked to base by radio. Finally, I made sure that all the students carried glucose and glucagon all the time, that all instructors and BDA staff carried solid and liquid glucose, glucagon and blood testing kit on their persons all the time, and that comprehensive medical supplies including intravenous fluids were readily available at base and in camp. Full first aid kits also went out with all groups away from base.

Why tell you all this?
Surely the idea of this book is to encourage people with diabetes to get out and do things? Why destroy the illusion that a group of teenagers with diabetes just went up to the Lake District and had a great time doing exciting things with no hassle about their diabetes? The point is that in order for people with diabetes to do anything like this there has to be some careful background planning. The reason that the diabetes did not get in the way for most of the participants is because of the background thought. Yes, I do believe that people with diabetes can do nearly anything they want provided they use common sense and are fully aware of the risks. When people with diabetes ask me if it is all right for them to try a potentially dangerous sport I suggest that they weigh the potential enjoyment and benefit against the risks to anyone doing the sport, and the risks to them as diabetics. If the risks are high, an activity is worth doing only if you desperately want or need to do it. If the only way out of a burning ship is to jump into the water, you have to jump. But if someone dares you to go parachute jumping and you are scared of heights and do not really want to, then do not do it.

The course

The BDA/OB mountain course is based at the OB centre in Eskdale with expeditions out into the mountains. Each day starts with a run and a dip into the tarn, followed by showers and breakfast. Sometimes the morning is spent on one activity, the afternoon on another, but some activities take one or two days. Further exercises fill the evenings. BDA staff live in the same accommodation as the students and share in all the activities.

Insulin or pills and food

When we started these courses no one knew what insulin reduction and food increase would be appropriate. Over the past ten years the participants and I have learned several lessons about insulin dose reduction and food increase. First, it is best to make the main insulin reduction and food increase on the first day of the course. This may mean that a few people have their blood glucose running a little high on the second day, but most have no problems. Second, the reduction in insulin dose needs to be greater than you would expect. Nowadays I advise students to reduce their insulin dose by 15 to 20 per cent of the pre-course level and by 30 to 50 per cent if they are prone to hypoglycaemic attacks at home. Experience has taught us that students who have ever had a hypoglycaemic eposide without warning or which they have been unable treat themselves they are at higher risk of hypoglycaemia than other people with diabetes. People on oral hypoglycaemic pills should reduce their pills by a third to a half, or if they are taking a very small dose, stop it altogether. At the same time I suggest that they double their snacks or increase their daily carbohydrate intake by about 50 g a day and gradually increase this during the course.

Morning routine

Many OB centres start the day with a jog and swim before breakfast. While this is no problem for people being treated by diet alone or pills, it is more difficult for those on insulin. When should you take the insulin? When and what should you eat? The main risk is of hypoglycaemia in the water when the run has used up your available energy. However, you do not want to eat something and then run on a full stomach. You also need some insulin to allow your muscles to use the energy you have just eaten. But if you have your insulin immediately before too small a snack you may go hypoglycaemic. This is more likely to occur if you have taken the insulin in your leg because exercise will increase the blood supply to this region and the insulin will be absorbed more rapidly.

The solution varies with the individual. If you tend to wake up low or

121

normal, have milk and biscuits or crackers and go for the jog and swim. Take your insulin on your return and then have breakfast. If you wake up with medium glucose levels, your insulin is probably running out, but practical experience suggests that you can manage a short jog and swim on a smaller snack, such as one biscuit or cracker, or possibly none. Take your insulin on your return. If you wake up high, your evening insulin has been used up. If you exercise, you run the risk of ketosis. You should have your insulin and a more substantial snack before you exercise, and try to sort out your evening food and insulin for next time (see the dawn phenomenon, page 51).

If you are only jogging and not leaping into cold water at the end of the run, you can keep your glucose level a little lower because you are not at risk of drowning if you go hypoglycaemic. However, you may be at risk of being knocked down in the road if you are running in town.

Rock sports
I once read in a textbook that people with diabetes should not go rock climbing. There is no reason why you should not enjoy rock sports provided you obey the safety rules. Rock climbers should use safety ropes and climbing belts or harnesses and learn to climb with a properly trained instructor. All equipment should be of a high standard and well maintained. Diabetic climbers should ensure that their blood glucose is at least 7 mmol/l (126 mg/dl) before starting a climb and eat a couple of glucose (dextrose) tablets immediately before climbing. They should have glucose tablets on their person where they can be reached easily with one hand and where they will not fall out. Your glucose will be no use if it is lying on the grass 60 feet below you! We use ski bags or bum bags with zippers to carry glucose for all activities on BDA/OB courses that are not on or in water (see the picture opposite).

Hypoglycaemia Signs of hypoglycaemia are unusual slowness, great difficulty finding hand or footholds or uncharacteristic irritation or fear. Sometimes it may lead to the diabetic climber becoming crag fast, when he is unable to move up or down. If any of these signs appear, the person controlling the safety rope (the belayer) should stop the rope (that is, fix it so that it cannot move) and insist that the climber has some glucose. If necessary, someone may need to go to the climber's assistance. Because of this, a diabetic should not go climbing in a group of fewer than three people.

Abseiling is another exciting rock sport. Used by rock climbers as a means of getting down a cliff or crag, it has now gained popularity among outdoor centres as an activity that can be enjoyed on its own. It is a controlled way of descending using a rope or rope and harness.

One of the most popular trips on some of the BDA/OB courses is the

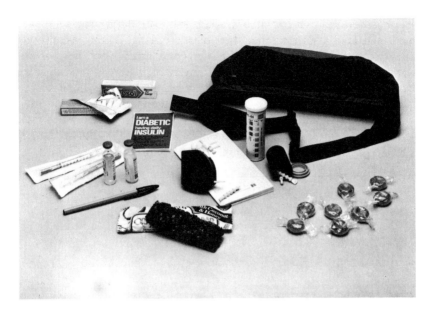

Diabetic kit for outdoor activities: bum bag with insulin and disposable syringes, blood glucose testing kit, diary and pen, 'sharps' container, diabetic card, glucose tablets and sweets or candy, and snack, for example, foil-wrapped high-fibre bars.

170-foot abseil down the sheer walls of an old slate quarry. A double abseil rope should be used so that if one rope shears there is a back-up. This is fed through a friction device, of which there are several types, and there is a separate safety rope. The abseiler controls the rate of descent by altering the angle of the abseil rope through the friction device. If he or she were to become unconscious and let go of the rope, gravity would take over and the descent would become virtually a free fall. A separately controlled safety rope protects the abseiler from this risk. The safety rope should always be attached to a climbing belt and at least a sit harness. Some instructors recommend a full body or alpine harness.

The feeling of triumph when you reach the top of a climb or the exhilaration of abseiling has to be experienced to be believed. So far, most of the students on BDA/OB courses have tried both, and many have chosen to tackle more difficult routes later in their courses.

I have only two reservations about climbing for people with diabetes. First, there can be no unroped or solo climbing. Not long ago I heard of an experienced diabetic climber who fell and died while climbing alone. My second reservation is over lead climbing, in which the climber seeks out the route protected by a safety rope from below. He or she

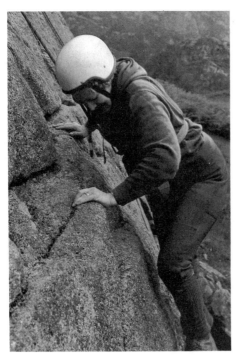

Rock climbing on one of the diabetics' Outward Bound courses – this is popular with all ages.

clips the rope through runners put in as he climbs. If he falls from above his last runner he descends twice that distance before being checked by the safety rope, and his safety depends on good, secure runners. This may mean a 20-foot fall if he is 10 feet above his last runner. The second climber is protected by a rope from above and the distance he falls is determined by the slack on the rope and the small amount if stretches (which should be only a few feet). Your diabetes must be very well-controlled, with good warning of hypoglycaemic attacks, and you must be a good climber, to lead.

Swimming
Outdoor swimming holds two risks for people with diabetes. One is the usual problem of coma due to hypoglycaemia, which may lead to drowning. The other is that of chilling, which may combine with mild hypoglycaemia to produce hypothermia, because someone who is hypoglycaemic cannot maintain his body temperature (see Chapter 11). People who have diabetes also tend to suffer from cramp more often than non-diabetics.

When swimming, you must have glucose on your person. Because glucose dissolves very easily, hard-boiled candy knotted into a plastic bag is more convenient. The plastic bag can be knotted around a safety pin attached to the bathing suit and torn open if needed. Small, well-sealed bottles of glucose gel (for example, Hypostop) are also useful kept in a pocket sewn into your swimming costume (see also Chapter 9).

Do not swim alone, and do not go out of your depth in unfamiliar water. Remember that swimming is physically demanding and that your blood glucose level may fall rapidly. Eat some glucose immediately before you get into the water. On BDA/OB courses no one is allowed to swim unless there is a qualified life saver on shore.

Canoeing
This is fun and can be as relaxing or as demanding as you want to make it. Always wear a life-jacket and carry hard-boiled glucose candy on your person, as I described for swimming.

One of the things that worries new canoeists is capsizing. Speaking as one who frequently capsizes, I assure you this is no problem. You simply fall out of the canoe and your life-jacket brings you safely to the surface. You will not get trapped in your canoe. Then your friends can, with practice, empty the canoe while you wait in the water and help you back into it – a deep

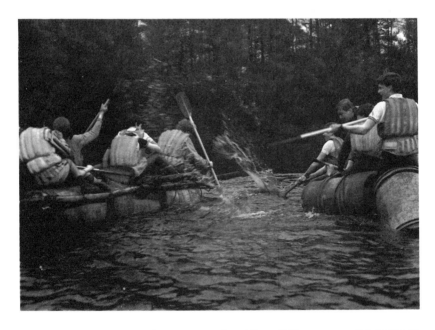

Raft racing proved one of the most enjoyable activities among the younger diabetic groups.

water rescue. With training, you can right the canoe with a rolling technique. Everyone who goes canoeing must do a carefully supervised practice capsize.

Beginners usually have difficulty steering the canoe and need to put a lot of effort into keeping it moving in a straight line. This means that they use a lot of energy and because of this we have frequent snack stops on the water. We all eat carbohydrate before going on the water. I usually ask everyone to check his or her blood glucose level before a canoeing session and anyone who is below 7 mmol/l (126 mg/dl) has an extra snack before going on the water. I started this procedure after seeing someone go from 7 to 2 mmol/l (126 to 36 mg/dl) after a quarter of an hour's canoeing. An instructor is always present during canoeing and resuscitation equipment is never more than a few minutes away.

Canoe trips need careful planning because the party will be away from roads and therefore emergency help for much of the time. There is not much space in a canoe and everything unprotected gets wet. All the participants carry their own snacks in plastic bags (at least twice the amount they would normally need) and the staff carry extra food in waterproof containers, and some drinking water. We also carry resuscitation equipment, spare woollen clothing, glucose and glucagon and a first aid kit, all in waterproof containers tied into the bottom of staff canoes. On meandering rivers it is especially important that the group stays together, to prevent the danger of someone having a hypoglycaemic attack around a corner out of sight. The staff are dispersed throughout the group, with the doctor at the back.

White-water canoeing requires a shore back-up and the groups have to be much smaller so that attention can be given to each person going over rough stretches.

You can get very cold on canoeing trips and warm clothes and windbreakers are essential. (Wool stays warm even when wet.) Wet suits should be worn in winter. Warm, dry clothes should be available at the destination to stop further chilling while you are packing up and loading the vehicle to return to base. Extra food should also be available in the vehicle.

Hypoglycaemia A capsize may be the first sign of a hypoglycaemic attack. Some people behave recklessly when going hypoglycaemic and capsize because of it. Others just drift farther and farther towards the back of the group as they get more and more tired. It is virtually impossible to decide if someone who has just found himself head first in the cold water is hypoglycaemic or not and so our rule is to give glucose after every capsize.

Ropes courses

All OB centres have a ropes course strung in the trees. Low obstacles are difficult, high ones easy. We run safety ropes over the high obstacles and the students clip themselves into these, moving from one safety rope to another without ever being unclipped altogether. Some of the obstacles are terrifying. It is difficult for a person with diabetes to decide whether the pounding heart, sweating and trembling is caused by fear or hypoglycaemia. This is because the same hormones that produce the symptoms of hypoglycaemia – adrenaline (epinephrine) and noradrenaline (norepinephrine) – are released by fear. The ropes course requires coordination and concentration and is not the place to have a hypoglycaemic attack. As with rock climbing, everyone eats one or two glucose tablets before starting on the ropes and wears a bum bag all the time.

Danny, a sixteen-year-old on insulin, who is a little absent-minded, was having difficulty on the 50-foot-long Burma rope bridge strung 20 feet in the air across the course.

Halfway across he said, in a rather small voice, 'I think I need some glucose.'

'Well, have some then!' I replied from below.

He pointed to the base of a tree 20 feet down where his bum bag was lying! I had to climb a tree in a hurry and meet him with some glucose.

As with other activities, the signs of hypoglycaemia are poor coordination, difficulty in doing something, or long periods of indecision. The main rule is not to move on and unclip from the safety rope you are on until your blood glucose level has been restored.

Night exercises

Most of us sleep at night. This means that we are not used to needing energy then. If you are running through a forest or building a bridge in the dark, you need lots to eat, perhaps a triple evening snack, and less evening insulin, perhaps 25 per cent less short-acting insulin.

The night exercises on the BDA/OB courses are very exciting and involve complicated problem solving and team work, for example, to rescue the damsel from the bandit chief in his stronghold in the forest. Teams have to stick together and everyone carries glucose. Staff use radios to keep in touch and track groups in the dark to ensure that everyone is accounted for. An extra snack is always available in the vehicle and back at base.

Orienteering

Map reading with pinpoint accuracy and speed are needed for orienteering. The object is to find markers on the mountain-side with clippers attached.

When you find the marker you clip your record sheet to it to prove that you have found it. We usually run this as a team event, with at least two students in each team, and more for younger groups. Because the fastest team to find all the markers is the winner, there is a tendency for students to ignore warning symptoms of hypoglycaemia deliberately so as not to hold the others in the group back. Then they have a bad hypoglycaemic attack on the mountain. The rule is, have large snacks before orienteering and take plenty to eat in the bum bags.

Staff usually monitor the progress of the teams from high vantage points. The most important one is the long stop at the end of the course, because at Eskdale poor navigators could end up on top of Scafell Pike (the highest mountain in England) if they were to get lost on the orienteering trail!

First aid and mountain rescue

OB centres in mountain areas provide mountain rescue teams. These teams are composed of instructors, backed-up by the students in the centre at that time if more manpower is needed, for example, for a search. Thus, the BDA/OB course students may be called on to help with rescues in Eskdale. Besides, since all participants go on mountain expeditions it is important that they know what to do if something goes wrong.

At first I started giving everyone basic first aid training. However, it rapidly became obvious that people with diabetes know a good deal more about first aid than non-diabetics of the same age. So later courses have had more advanced first aid training. Participants go on exercises to solve all types of difficult problems, such as what to do with the fallen climber or the hypothermic camper, and they cope very well.

To start with, first aid and rescue sessions take place on the campus. As groups become more experienced they are given search and rescue exercises in the mountains. They set off with one or two stretchers and locate the casualty, usually the long-suffering medical officer or nurse, made up with dramatic injuries. They are also often hampered in their efforts by a 'hysterical friend' who gets in the way and has to be rescued too. The rescue usually culminates in a stretcher being lowered over a cliff, which needs team work and coordination from the participants and steady nerves on the part of the casualty. These exercises may start off as a game but they rapidly become serious as students realize that they are taking responsibility for the casualty's life, actor or not. Obviously, all the exercises are supervised by instructors.

If someone with diabetes has an accident in the mountains all the usual first aid principles apply: maintenance of airway, breathing and circulation, stopping bleeding, and ensuring that an unconscious person cannot inhale vomit or other material. Obviously, the casualty must be carefully assessed, treated for injuries and protected from further harm while mountain rescue procedures are put into effect and help is sought. The additional factor with a diabetic casualty is the blood glucose level. This should be measured at hourly intervals and written down in the record you are keeping for the rescue services. If the glucose is below 3.5 mmol/l (63 mg/dl), oral glucose should be given. Glucose can be swallowed by a conscious casualty and rubbed inside the mouth of an unconscious one. Record the amount of food or drink given to the casualty and the time at which it was given. Hot, sweet tea may be especially helpful in cold weather. It may take many hours for help to arrive, but in situations where help can arrive fast and there is no risk of hypoglycaemia do not give the injured person anything to eat or drink. Normally one should not feed anyone who has been injured as it could cause problems if they need an anaesthetic. If the casualty's glucose level is above 13 mmol/l (234 mg/dl) give 2 units of rapid-acting insulin, intramuscularly, so that it is better absorbed. This can be repeated hourly if indicated.

Responsibility   Team work and shared responsibility are an important part of these OB courses. Each student is there as an individual to try new activities and overcome personal challenges, but the participants are also part of a group and are expected to keep an eye out for each other. It is rare for BDA staff to have to treat hypoglycaemic attacks. Generally fellow students deal with them at the first sign that all is not well. Students teach each other how to monitor blood glucose levels and all sorts of new tricks with injection techniques and diabetic problem solving. As the course progresses they take a pride in sorting themselves out. Weaker students are supervised by more able ones, with continuous encouragement and support. Many of the activities are team challenges with everyone in the group contributing. The idea of taking responsibility for other people may come strangely to a young person who has been diabetic for a long time. Generally, the person with diabetes is the one who is looked after. Yet because of this, people with diabetes are good at looking after other people and are sensitive to their needs.

Mountain expeditions

The mountains are the place where I recharge my batteries. After the toil of a steep walk you stand on the summit with the fresh wind on your face, looking out over mile upon mile of hills and valleys, to the endless sky with its sweeping clouds and changing lights.

Mountains are places of beauty, and most of their beauties are not hard to reach, requiring just a little effort and energy. But this ease of access belies their need to be treated with respect. Every year people die in the mountains, usually because they underestimated the potential dangers. The most important safety rule is to assume that the worst may happen and then work out how you can prevent it or cope with it. You must be able to cope with getting lost, staying out all night, someone becoming ill or injured, getting too cold, too wet, too hot or too dry.

National mountaineering organizations will give you specfic advice about walking in your area. Ask for it and follow it. They know – they are the ones who rescue people who have not asked for advice. This chapter gives additional advice for diabetic individuals or groups. If none of you is experienced in mountain walking it is best to find someone who is to help you. A large group of people with diabetes on anything other than a short walk should have an accompanying doctor. BDA/OB course groups are accompanied by BDA and OB staff on their first expeditions and shadowed by staff (who only intervene in emergencies) on subsequent expeditions.

Safety in numbers, with good equipment If you cannot read a map, learn how to do it or go with someone who can. The minimum size for a party is four – one person to stay with a casualty and two to go for help. The party always travel together, moving at the speed of the slowest person.

Wear good walking boots and make sure that they do not rub your feet. Wear clothing appropriate to the area you are going to and the time of year, and carry windproof and waterproof clothes whatever the weather. Sun in the valley is not incompatible with pouring rain and howling gales on the mountain tops. The party should carry adequate overnight shelter for an emergency and the means to keep themselves warm in the shelter (for example, a tent and two sleeping bags for four people). They should also carry a stove and fuel. Everyone should have a map, compass and whistle, and know what to do with them.

Diabetic travel pack and food Each of the diabetics should carry his own diabetic travel pack (see page 134), twice as much food as he expects to eat for meals, six double snacks and emergency glucose. As a rough guide we use the MBE – Mars Bar Equivalent – for snacks (based on the standard size Mars Bar). Diabetic walkers should learn to eat as they travel, and remember that they need to travel slowly in the mountains because of this need for frequent snack stops. If you are in a diabetic group inexperienced in mountain walking, add at least an hour for every three you have calculated from distance and ascent that the journey will take.

The continuous exercise of mountain walking uses up a lot of energy and it is very important that you do not become hypoglycaemic. The group leader should stay at the back of the group to pick up people who have slowed down because of hypoglycaemic attacks or other problems, and make sure that no one gets left behind. I have been astonished by the quantity of food that some students need to eat when out on an expedition.

Seventeen-year-old Bill, on twice-daily insulin – which he had reduced by 20 per cent – led a group of six people with diabetes over a steep ten mile route in the mountains. During the day he ate a huge breakfast, lunch and evening meal (each about double his usual calorie and carbohydrate content), seven Mars bars, six high fibre bars, a packet of glucose tablets and three apples. His blood glucose before bed that evening was 4 mmol/l (72 mg/dl).

Water   If clean water is not readily available the group will also need to carry some. This is especially important in very hot weather as a large amount of fluid is lost as sweat, and dehydration can occur; I have had to treat heat stroke in the Lake District in Britain (in a non-diabetic). In very hot weather your food should also be very salty because salt is lost in sweat. People with diabetes are prone to cramp and need plenty of salt to replace what is lost by sweating. Quinine-containing drinks such as bitter lemon or tonic may help.

Hypothermia   The dangers of hypothermia and hypoglycaemia which I discuss in Chapter 11 are especially applicable here.

Janine (whom we met in Chapter 5) suddenly became unconscious from hypoglycaemia while eating her lunch after a cold, wet, windy mountain walk. She rapidly became very cold. She was revived by glucose rubbed inside her mouth, started shivering and then regained consciousness. It took some time to warm her in a sleeping bag with another group member and hot, sweet drinks.

Hypoglycaemia and ketoacidosis   Hypoglycaemia can be recognized by someone stumbling, slowing down, getting muddled about navigation, showing sudden exhaustion, argumentativeness or suddenly losing consciousness. Many people with diabetes, who are not used to walking long distances lose their ability to distinguish between tiredness and hypoglycaemia. If you are tired, eat something. A word of warning – you can overdo the eating. Obviously, you can check your blood glucose if you are not sure whether you are tired or hypoglycaemic.

Prolonged exercise make ketosis worse. If you have high or moderately high blood glucose levels, or have not been feeling very well, check your urine for ketones. If you have moderate or heavy ketones do not go on an expedition. You may develop ketoacidosis and then you will be a danger to yourself and your friends. You need more insulin and should not exercise heavily until you have got rid of the ketones. As a general principle, if you are not well, stay at home. It is not fair to saddle your friends with someone who may collapse on top of a mountain many hours away from the nearest telephone. They are morally obliged to help you and they may be put at risk trying to sort you out.

Camping

The amount of equipment you need varies depending on where you are planning to camp, the time of year, how far you have to carry the gear and how long you intend to stay there. Again, your national mountaineering council can advise you.

You will need your diabetes travel pack and plenty of food. Do your calculations properly beforehand, and as with all expeditions, take twice as much food as you expect to eat because some may get spoiled, or you may get stuck somewhere. Make sure that you have a good supply of clean water. Remember that camp cooking takes longer than home cooking and it is difficult to predict when a meal will be ready. Either have a cold first course, for example, bread and margarine, or do not take your insulin until your food is ready to eat.

Diabetic campers should not sleep alone. You will probably be combining camping with an active vacation and will therefore be at risk of nocturnal hypoglycaemia. The group leader should check all the tents after supper to make sure that everyone has eaten and is all right.

Always bear these points in mind:

- People with diabetes can enjoy an OB mountain course without their diabetes getting in their way and without losing control of their blood glucose levels.
- If you want to try new outdoor activities, learn from properly qualified instructors.
- When planning new activities assume that the worst will happen and then plan how to prevent it or cope with it if it happens (it very rarely does).
- Always obey safety rules absolutely.
- Use the right equipment, properly maintained, and the right clothing.
- Seek expert local advice.
- Make certain that you will not go hypoglycaemic. Always carry glucose on your person where it cannot get lost and can be reached with one hand in any position. Reduce your insulin or pills and increase your food. Always carry twice the amount of food you think you will need as well as your travel pack.

- Do not do it alone.
- Weigh the benefits and pleasures of a planned activity against the risks.
- Have fun!

11 Travel

As a person with diabetes who has conquered its problems, you may well be doing a fair amount of travelling both for work and pleasure. The practicalities of travel frequently worry people with diabetes. What if there is a traffic jam? Will I be able to get a meal when I get there? What will I do if the flight is delayed? How do I cope with time zones? What if I am seasick? There are further concerns about driving. Am I fit to drive? What are the legal problems concerned with driving? The message, as usual, is to think about potential problems beforehand and be prepared.

The diabetes travel pack
You should carry the following in a robust waterproof bag or wallet:

1. Your diabetic card with help telephone number
2. A card in the language of the country or countries you are visiting, explaining that you have diabetes and saying what to do if you have a hypoglycaemic attack
3. Any documents you need for reciprocal health agreements or health insurance
4. Blood and/or urine glucose testing kit
5. Ketone testing kit
6. Insulin (two bottles of each type) – or pen cartridges
7. Disposable syringes and needles – or your insulin pen
8. Foil-wrapped alcohol swabs
9. Oral hypoglycaemic pills
10. Paper tissues
11. Baby wipes or other prepacked skin cleaners
12. Motion sickness pills
13. First aid kit
14. Something to put sharps into
15. Some glucose and hard-boiled glucose candy.

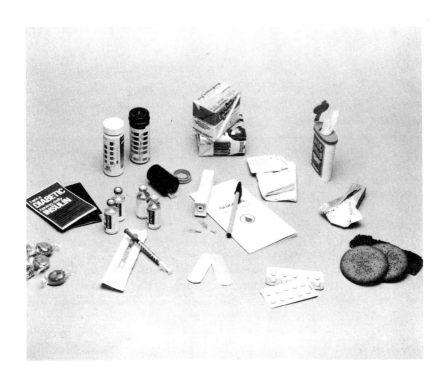

The diabetes travel pack: diabetic card, foreign language diabetic card and health documents, blood glucose testing kit, 'sharps' container, urine glucose and ketone testing strips, insulin and disposable syringes, oral hypoglycaemic pills, foil-wrapped alcohol swabs, prepacked moist skin cleaner, paper tissues, motion sickness pills, sticking plaster (plus personal first aid kit – not shown), glucose tablets and boiled glucose sweets or candy, fruit juice, biscuits or cookies, high-fibre bars.

This will all fit into a small ski or bum bag. You should also carry a leak-proof bottle of plain water, cans or cartons of fruit juice, and snacks.

The diabetes travel pack should be with you in a bum bag or shoulder bag and be carried all the time. You will also need to take food for twice the number of meals you expect to need. A further supply of insulin or pills should be carried in other luggage in case you lose your diabetes travel pack. Your travelling companion could carry the spare supply if you wish, and in any case should always carry glucose. It is also a good idea for your companion to carry glucagon. Novo Nordisk (UK) make an 'all-in-one-pack' including glucagon, syringe and needle.

Driving
The law   The legal requirements for driving differ in different countries,

but most insist that you notify them of any illness that may impair your safety as a driver. For example, the old British driving licence states:

> You are required by law to inform Driver and Vehicle Licensing Centre (DVLC) . . . at once if you have any disability which is or may become likely to affect your fitness as a driver, unless you do not expect it to last for more than 3 months.

The new licence mentions diabetes specifically. The DVLC is now the DVLA. Drug-treated diabetes counts as such a disability because people on drugs which lower the blood glucose (this includes insulin) are at risk of hypoglycaemia and confusion or coma. It can be argued that any form of diabetes counts because of the theoretical risk of hyperglycaemic como, or the later need for glucose lowering treatment, or because some of the complications of diabetes may make driving unsafe. To adhere to the letter of the law, even diet-treated diabetics should inform the DVLA of their diagnosis, clearly stating that they are not taking blood glucose lowering drugs at that time.

It is your responsibility to notify the authorities and not your doctor's. The licensing authority may then request details of your condition from your doctor who can release them only with your consent.

Car insurance You must also tell your car insurance company that you have diabetes. Again, this responsibility is yours. It is silly not to tell them, because if you make a claim and have not revealed your diabetes they may refuse to pay, whether the accident was your fault or not. They may also refuse to pay if you have not told the licensing authority.

Driving with diabetes is not simply a matter of getting official approval. It is important that you and other road users are completely safe. What factors should be considered if you want to drive a car? First, are you at any risk of becoming confused or unconscious? Never drive any vehicle if your blood glucose is below 4 mmol/l (72 mg/dl) or if you feel hypoglycaemic.

If you need to make a journey just before a meal, eat a snack before you get into the car. You must have glucose in the car, and you should have enough food in the car for an extra meal in case of breakdowns or delays. Some people with diabetes who do a lot of travelling, carry their diabetes travel pack in the car all the time in case they need to spend a night away from home.

If you feel at all hypoglycaemic while you are driving, stop as soon as it is safe to do so, turn off the engine and remove the ignition keys. Then have something to eat. You should also slide into the passenger seat so that you are not 'in control of the vehicle'. Remember that you may not be thinking straight or be properly coordinated if you are hypoglycaemic. I heard of one man who drove five miles while hypoglycaemic and left a trail of destruction throughout the entire length of a village street.

Next, you should consider whether you have any complications of diabetes which may make driving hazardous. An obvious one is diabetic retinopathy (see also Chapter 4). Most people with retinopathy can see well enough to drive but it is important that you have your visual acuity and your visual field (all round vision) checked regularly. If you have had a lot of photocoagulation your visual field may be narrower than before. If you have maculopathy (damage to the area of best vision) you may not be able to see well enough to drive. Cataracts may also block your vision for driving and this may be an added reason to have them removed.

If you have numb hands or feet from diabetic neuropathy you may not be able to feel the controls of the car very well; and if you have heart trouble, you should discuss driving with your doctor. The current advice is that you should not drive for at least one month after a heart attack. If you have angina that may be brought on by stress, such as road hogs and traffic jams, you should certainly not drive.

Travel by bus or rail

The main problem with bus journeys is keeping comfortable. Otherwise, once you have got on to a bus all you have to do is sit down until you reach your destination. Not all buses have lavatories so it is a good idea to make sure your blood glucose is below your renal threshold during the journey. You will, of course need your diabetes travel pack.

Most trains in the developed countries have lavatories but there may be none in Third World countries. Again you will need to make sure your blood glucose is below your renal threshold. If you are travelling in an out of the way place, you will also need a far larger food and fluid reserve, and should plan your trip more as I described for mountain expeditions (see Chapter 10).

Travel by sea

If you know you are a bad sailor, take a motion sickness pill before you step on board ship and keep taking them at the interval stated on the package until you are safely on dry land again. These pills, of which a range are available from pharmacies, drugstores or doctors, will not upset your diabetes, but sea sickness might. The pills may make you drowsy, though, and so you should not take them if, for example, you are planning to drive your car off the ferry.

What should you do if sea sickness strikes? Try to find somewhere to lie down with some fresh air. Ask a steward for a motion sickness pill if you do not have any. Check your blood glucose level every couple of hours and suck some glucose tablets or have a glucose drink such as Lucozade if it is low. Take a few units of rapid-acting insulin every four hours if your blood glucose level is high. This is unlikely because motion sickness is not usually related to a generalized infection, like gastroenteritis, and so there is no increase in insulin resistance. Your glucose level will tend to go down in most cases. You may feel as if you want to die while you are sea sick, but you will recover quickly when you are back on land.

Travel by air
Air travel has several special problems for the person with insulin-treated (and, to some extent, the non-insulin-treated) diabetes:

1. You are at the mercy of the airline and their timetable
2. Your luggage is restricted
3. You are more likely to have trouble with customs checks
4. You may travel rapidly through time zones.

Unpredictability   The first problem is simply that of the unpredictability of air travel. Your diabetes travel pack and extra food should see you through this, and besides you will usually be able to buy food and drink at the airport. Your main luggage will be taken from you and put in the hold, where it may be frozen in flight. You must, therefore, have all your insulin with you inside the passenger compartment as it is destroyed by freezing. You must keep your diabetes travel pack with you.

Customs   Customs officers and airline officials using x-ray scanners frequently stop people with diabetes because syringes and needles show up on their screens. This is why you need your diabetic card and an explanation of it in the language of the country you are visiting. There should be no problem, once you have explained the situation, so do not get angry or upset.

Time zones   Adjustment from home time to foreign time is complicated. *If you are taking oral hypoglycaemic pills*, work out the total dose of pills you take in twenty-four hours. Next consider the actual number of hours between breakfast on the day you leave home and the first breakfast in the country you are visiting. By breakfast, I mean the meal eaten on getting up in the morning, whatever it is called locally. If there are twenty-four hours or more between these two breakfasts take your total twenty-four hour dose of pills split at appropriate intervals. Do not take more than this, but wait until your first breakfast in your new country before you start taking your pills during the day as you would at home. If there are less than twenty-four hours between your breakfast at home and your first breakfast in your new country, take fewer pills. Thus, if there are twelve hours, take half your pills, eighteen hours, two-thirds of your pills and so on. You will need to use a bit of common sense to arrive at a practical division. Follow a similar process on the way home.

If you are taking insulin you can use the same calculation if you wish, but their type of insulin and its duration of action has to be considered. The main concern is not to have a hypoglycaemic attack in some remote corner of a foreign airport. This is not a hypothetical worry. You are tired and the food on the aeroplane was indigestible; you may have had a couple of free drinks, you have lugged two suitcases, a shoulder bag, two carriers of duty free wine and a souvenir from Barcelona through endless miles of corridors; your next flight has just been delayed for four hours and the restaurant is shut. As always, check your blood glucose and do not care if anyone sees you.

How do you calculate your insulin? *If you are on one injection of very long-acting insulin a day and two or more injections of rapid-acting insulin*: Calculate the number of actual hours between breakfast at home and your first breakfast in the new country. If this is twenty-four hours or more, take your usual dose of very long-acting insulin; if less than this, take an appropriate proportion (for example, for twelve hours half the dose, twenty hours 80 per cent of the dose and so on). Take your usual short-acting insulin before breakfast at home and then check your blood glucose levels before each meal you have until the first breakfast. If they are 7 mmol/l or more (126 mg/dl) take 2 to 4 units of rapid-acting insulin to cover each meal. If they are below 4 mmol/l (72 mg/dl), eat a bigger meal and start it with some fast-acting carbohydrate. Before breakfast in the new country have your usual insulin and continue this, with frequent blood glucose measurements and adjustments as necessary, until you come home. Then follow a similar process when you arrive home.

If you are on two injections of medium-acting or long-acting insulin with short-acting insulin a day: twenty-four hours or more between your home breakfast and your next breakfast, take your usual insulin before breakfast at home and twelve hours later (or at the meal nearest to twelve hours later) take your 'evening' dose. It may be wise to reduce each dose by a small proportion, for example, 10 per cent, to make sure that you do not go hypoglycaemic. Then have your usual insulin before the next breakfast as above.

Less than twenty-four hours between the two breakfasts, take your usual insulin before breakfast at home (reduced a little if you wish). Then take no more long-acting or medium-acting insulin until the next breakfast. Check your blood glucose level before each main meal and give 2 to 4 units of insulin if it is 7 mmol/l or more. Have your usual medium-acting or long-acting and fast-acting insulin before your first breakfast in the new country. Reverse the process for your return trip.

This advice can be modified by your personal experience. If you make

Travel by air – two examples of diabetes management

Peter: New York by Concorde to London

Usual insulin: Actrapid (short acting) 8 u am, 6 u pm
Ultratard (very long acting) 20 u am

New York Time, hrs	London Time, hrs	Blood glucose mmol/l (mg/dl)	Insulin	Food
07.00		7 (126)	Actrapid 6 u Ultratard 16 u	Meal
08.00				
09.00	Depart			Snack
10.00				
11.00	Flight	10 (180)	Actrapid 4 u	Meal
12.00				
13.00	Arrive 18.00			Snack
	19.00			
	20.00	7 (126)	Actrapid 6 u	Meal
	21.00			
	22.00			
	23.00	7 (126)		Snack
	Bed			
	07.00	4 (72)	Actrapid 8 u Ultratard 20 u	Meal

Breakfast to breakfast = 19 hrs, 19/24 = 80%

If Pete had been on oral hypoglycaemic pills, for example, glibenclamide 10 mg pre-breakfast, 5 mg pre-evening meal, I would have suggested 80% of 15 mg = 12.5 mg total dose as 7.5 mg pre-breakfast. 5 mg pre-evening meal.

Mary: London to Vancouver

Usual insulin: Velosulin (short acting) 12 u am, 8 u pm
           Insulatard (medium acting) 20 u am, 16 u pm

London Time, hrs	Vancouver Time, hrs	Blood glucose mmol/l (mg/dl)	Insulin	Food
07.00		7 (126)	Velosulin 12 u Insulatard 18 u	Meal
08.00				
09.00				
10.00				Snack
11.00				
12.00		4 (72)	—	Meal
13.00	Depart			
14.00				
15.00				Snack
16.00				
17.00	Flight	10 (180)	Velosulin 4 u	Meal
18.00			Insulatard 12u	
19.00				Snack
20.00				
21.00		7 (126)	Velosulin 4 u	Meal
22.00	Arrive			
	14.00			
	15.00			Snack
	16.00			
	17.00			
	18.00	4 (72)	—	Meal
	19.00			
	20.00			
	21.00	7 (126)	Velosulin 2 u	Snack
	22.00			
	Bed			
	07.00	10 (180)	Velosulin 12 u Insulatard 20 u	Meal

Breakfast to breakfast 32 hrs

regular trips across a particular time zone, you should be able to work out your best insulin dose from experience. What I have suggested may cause you to run your blood glucose level a little high for the first few days, but that is better than going hypoglycaemic in a strange country.

Very long trips If you are on a very long trip, of more than thirty-six hours, divide the journey into 'night' (sleeping time) and 'day', and have three meals and your usual between meal snacks during the 'day'. Have a slightly reduced dose of your insulin as usual before the first meal after waking and before the last meal before sleeping. Check your blood glucose level before each meal and before bed and if it is high, top up with 2 to 4 units of fast-acting insulin. It is better to err towards 10 mmol/l (180 mg/dl) than 4 mmol/l (72 mg/dl) when travelling, to make sure that you avoid hypoglycaemic attacks.

Funny foreign food

There is no reason why people with diabetes should not be adventurous in their eating. Avoid obviously sugary or very greasy foods. Fresh food (providing it is well washed or cooked) is usually all right. Fish is a good food for a diabetic diet. Pasta (sometimes the wholewheat variety) and rice are available in most places, and many different countries use beans and legumes in their cooking. If a strange dish looks tempting, try it – the occasional naughty food is not a disaster. If the meals are larger than you are used to, have a little more rapid-acting insulin before them.

If the meal times are very different from those at home, do not worry. If you are on once-daily very long-acting and several rapid-acting doses of insulin, have your rapid-acting insulin before the meal, whenever it is. If you are on twice-daily medium-acting or long-acting with short-acting insulin, you can either take both the medium-acting or long-acting and short-acting insulin before the evening meal whenever that is, or, if this is going to create problems overnight, take your medium-acting or long-acting insulin at the usual time and have the rapid-acting insulin before the evening meal. Consider the interval between injections and try to ensure that the medium-acting and long-acting injections are spaced out, as they would be at home. Your changed eating habits are only for a limited period.

However, you should not forget to adjust your insulin dose and food intake to suit your level of activity. Lying in the sun uses up less energy than tramping around ancient monuments.

Traveller's tummy

Some people are unlucky enough to develop diarrhoea and vomiting while on holiday. For this reason, it is a good idea to ask your doctor to give you some anti-emetic and anti-diarrhoeal pills to take with you. At the first sign of trouble get yourself to a comfortable refuge with a bed and a toilet. Get a

142

large supply of clean water – mineral water in sealed bottles is safe – and some liquid glucose such as Lucozade, Coca Cola or Pepsi Cola. Start checking your blood glucose level and proceed as described in Chapter 3. Your glucose level will probably rise and you may need more insulin than usual. Be prepared to check your glucose very frequently, probably every one or two hours, if things start to go very awry, and take more frequent additional doses of fast-acting insulin. Get help early if needed.

If you are on oral hypoglycaemic pills you may vomit them up or not absorb them because of the diarrhoea. If you see recognizable pills in the vomit, try taking some more pills at the same dose. If they still do not stay down, or your glucose level starts to rise, you probably need some insulin to tide you over the attack. Seek medical help.

If you are vomiting and not managing to eat you may start making starvation ketones. If your glucose is low, try sipping your sugary drink, because even if you vomit you will have absorbed some glucose through your mouth. Alternatively, try sucking glucose tablets. When you feel like eating a little, try a few digestive biscuits, Graham crackers or something similar. During a diarrhoeal illness you may lose a lot of fluid and in some cases this may make you feel lightheaded. This may be more pronounced if you have autonomic neuropathy. Try to keep drinking small amounts of fluid all the time, to keep up with what you are losing. If you feel giddy, get up slowly, and call a doctor. When the worst is over, give yourself a day or two to recover gently.

Illness
People with diabetes who keep an eye on themselves and use some common sense are no more likely to get ill abroad than anyone else. However, a little forward planning is prudent. Before going away, take out travel insurance. Make sure that it is the type that will cover hospital and medical expenses in the country you are visiting and that if necessary it will cover the cost of your being flown home with a medical escort. If you are planning to spend a long time in a foreign country your doctor may be able to give you the name of a local diabetologist (the International Diabetes Federation has members in virtually every country in the world).

It may be useful to carry with you a letter summarizing your medical condition and medication. If you need medical help, try to find a doctor who speaks your language and make certain that he knows that you are diabetic and that you need insulin or tablets (hang on to your personal supply in case the doctor or hospital do not have that brand, and ask what dose to take). If you get very ill in a remote part of the world it may be better to be flown home, assuming that the pressure changes of air travel are not hazardous for your condition.

Temperature

Heat   Hot sun and exercise may increase the rate of absorption of your insulin. Very hot weather may lead to dehydration and may increase the effects of urine loss associated with a raised blood glucose. It is important to drink plenty of fluids. Beware sunburn.

Cold   Intense cold may mean that your insulin is absorbed slowly to start with and then is rapidly absorbed later when you warm up by the fire or in a warm bath. If you are out in cold, wet or windy conditions for any length of time, make sure that you are well protected against both wind and wet. The advice I gave in Chapters 9 and 10 on clothing and equipment for energetic expeditions is useful for all trips of this type.

People with diabetes who become chilled and hypoglycaemic are at special risk of severe hypothermia; and from that you can die, as has been made so clear from recent publicity about the aged, who are also at risk. Studies made in Nottingham, England, showed that if people are put in a very cold room their temperature begins to fall and they start to shiver as they try to keep warm. If they are then made hypoglycaemic they stop shivering and their body temperature plummets to dangerously low levels. As soon as their blood glucose is returned to normal, they start shivering again and the fall in body temperature is halted.

Always bear the following points in mind:

- Think ahead. Take out travel insurance. Always carry your diabetes travel pack on your person. Always take twice the number of meals you think you are going to need on a journey.
- Make sure that you are at no risk of hypoglycaemia when driving or travelling in a car. Tell the driver and vehicle licensing authorities and your insurance company that you are diabetic.
- Do not run the risk of hypoglycaemia in a strange town or country.
- Take motion sickness pills if you suspect you may need them and carry anti-emetics and anti-diarrhoeal pills.
- Plan any air trips carefully. Never allow your insulin to get frozen in the baggage compartment.
- Adjust your insulin to the way of life of the country you are visiting. Feel free to explore foreign food. If you get ill, start checking your glucose level frequently and adjust your treatment accordingly.
- Beware extremes of heat and cold.
- Learn from your experiences.
- Have a good trip!

12 Living with your diabetes

Doctors and other health care professionals talk about you as 'a diabetic' or 'a person with diabetes' and you may also talk about being a diabetic or having diabetes. But this is a very poor description of you. You are a unique individual with your own lifestyle, work, hobbies, family background, home, friends, ideas and dreams. No one else in the world is capable of offering your special gifts to society. The fact that you have, at some stage in your life, been diagnosed as having diabetes is a very small part of your whole person.

Your diabetes is also unique to you – no one else responds in precisely your way to changes in food, exercise, treatment and the passage of time. This is why it is very important that you learn all you can about your own diabetes. Armed with this knowledge and with the experience built up by health care professionals, scientists and others (including those with diabetes) you can take command of your diabetes and ensure that it remains well controlled and does not get in your way. Your diabetes is an inescapable part of you, but there is no need for it to intrude on your enjoyment of life.

This all sounds great in theory, but when you wake up in the middle of the night and start worrying and wish that it wasn't you, that it was all a terrible mistake and you are going to wake up in the morning undiabetic, then it is not so simple. Being diabetic is not easy all the time – there would be no need for this book if it were. The first, and maybe the hardest, step is to accept that you have diabetes and that for the forseeable future you will remain so. This acceptance does not come overnight and some people with diabetes never fully accept it.

Jo has been diabetic for ten of her eighteen years. Nowadays she is in and out of hospital with ketoacidosis and mistakes in her insulin dose. I asked her how she felt about being diabetic and the answer was simple: 'I don't want to know.'

145

Being an ostrich is all very well, but if you try to bury your diabetes in the sand you find that the rest of you gets covered in grit too!

Give yourself a chance and do not expect too much of yourself all at once. If you are reading this book you should not be a beginner, but even experienced diabetics may find they need to think about some parts of it.

There is a tendency to see diabetes in terms of blood glucose levels and the mechanics of insulin injection or pill dose. When you go to your clinic you will be asked all about this and about symptoms of tissue damage. Sadly, in many clinics, there is too little time and too clinical an atmosphere to discuss how you feel emotionally. Many people with diabetes feel that the doctor '. . . doesn't want to know about my private worries. He is much too busy thinking about my sugar levels.' If you are worried, then we do want to know. It will help us to help you, and you may feel better sharing your anxieties. If something is worrying you, even if it seems to be nothing to do with your diabetes, the anxiety may upset your glucose balance.

Nellie is seventy-five years old and has been diabetic for twenty years. When she came to the clinic recently she looked tired and had lost weight. I asked her how she was sleeping.

'I can hardly sleep at all. I'm so worried,' she said and she started crying quietly.

She told me that because her husband had worked past the official retirement age his pension had been reduced. They were finding it very hard to pay the bills and she could not afford her proper diet.

'But I'm keeping you from your work, doctor,' she said.

I pointed out that she was my work at the moment.

Later, I arranged for her to discuss things with our welfare expert, who found that she was entitled to an additional allowance.

Feel free to discuss how you view your diabetes with your diabetes advisers, your family doctor, your relatives and with your close friends. It will help them to understand. You will be helping your doctor too. I am not diabetic and I do not know what it feels like to have diabetes. I need my patients to tell me how they feel. I learn more from my patients than I ever have from textbooks, and that helps me to look after future patients.

Your diabetic adviser

The diagnosis of diabetes is made under many different circumstances, for example, during a routine medical examination for insurance purposes or during out-patient or in-patient care for other conditions; but most people first learn that they may have diabetes from their family doctor. What happens next varies. Some family doctors continue to provide all aspects of care for their diabetic patients, others refer them to a specialist with an interest in diabetes working on his own or within a hospital clinic. Some family doctors share the care of their diabetic patients with hospital diabetologists, or run their own mini-clinics.

Even if you are looked after by a diabetologist, it is still important that your family doctor knows what is going on as far as your diabetes is concerned. In Britain, and in many other countries, it is the family doctor who is called to your home in the middle of the night when you feel ill, whether your diabetes is the cause of your symptoms or not. Your family doctor cannot look after you properly if he or she does not have all your health details. Most diabetologists or diabetic clinics write to the family doctor every time a patient is seen. Some have cooperation cards kept by the patient on which clinical and laboratory details are written at each visit. If you have such a card, make sure that it is kept up to date and keep it safe and easy to find. If you have out-patient record cards of any sort, keep them where you can find them easily and take them with you whenever you see any doctor, or if you have to be admitted to the hospital.

Whatever arrangement you follow for your diabetic care, it is important that you and those caring for your health are clear who your diabetes adviser is. You must know who you should contact if you need help. You also need to know how to do this during office hours and at night or weekends. If you are unsure about this, clarify it with your family doctor and your diabetologist (if applicable) immediately. You should have on your diabetic card the name, address and telephone number of the person to be contacted in an emergency. Do not wait until three o'clock in the morning on a national holiday to find you have not got them.

When you first discovered that you have diabetes you needed a lot of help and advice. As you became more independent and confident, your contacts with your adviser probably became less frequent. You may have lost touch altogether. But no one ever stops learning about diabetes and even the most careful and expert people with diabetes occasionally need help. It is important that wherever you are, there is a doctor or diabetes specialist nurse whom you can contact if you are having difficulties, or for regular reviews.

You and your adviser may be together for many years, so it is important that you build up a trust and are able to get along reasonably well. Medical and paramedical staff are human and vary in their attitudes and their approach to problem solving and patient care. One doctor's manner and personality may suit one person but not another. It takes time for you to get to know your adviser and for him or her to get to know you. If, after a time, you really feel that you are not getting along, discuss your feelings with him or consider asking if you can see someone else.

Another factor that may influence your choice of adviser is the framework within which he works. For example, some people prefer to be

147

seen in small local centres, others like to go to large teaching centres. Some just like to see the doctor, others to see all the different specialized members of the health care team. You may not be able to choose exactly what you want, especially in country areas, but if you are unhappy with any aspect of your care and do not ask whether there is an alternative you will never find out about it!

Whatever you decide to do, you should be seen regularly by someone who checks up on your glucose balance, your diabetes and your general health. Diabetes is so common that there should be a doctor with this special interest near you. If you have no family doctor or have just moved to a new area, ask your local diabetic association for a list of doctors' names and clinics. Better still, if you are moving, ask your previous adviser to contact someone they know in your new area.

In the 1980's the department in which I worked arranged special clinic sessions to convert everyone taking insulin in the Oxford area to the U100 strength. Because pharmacists notified us of every diabetic for whom they filled a prescription for insulin, we discovered a group of people on insulin who had not been attending the clinic. They gave various reasons for not attending: some had moved, others were too busy, or had missed an appointment and not received another, or not sought one. Some of these people had severe diabetic tissue damage. If you miss an appointment, do not expect another to appear automatically. Most clinics and diabetes centres chase up non-attenders but notification of your appointment may have got lost in the mail or you may have forgotten to tell the clinic your new address. If you do not get a follow-up appointment, write or telephone and ask for another, or ask your family doctor to do this for you. Do not wait for five years wondering why nothing is happening – or put it off until tomorrow.

Some aspects of diabetes require special care, for example, pregnancy, proliferative retinopathy and renal disease. If this applies to you, your diabetes adviser will be able to tell you if this is one of his or her specialties; if not, he will arrange for you to see someone who is expert in this field. It is worth being prepared to travel to another city for expert care. Your diabetes adviser may also ask for a colleague's help if you have other forms of tissue damage such as peripheral vascular disease or heart trouble (see also Chapter 4).

Most people find going to doctors, clinics and hospitals worrying and there is a natural tendency to sit quietly and just do as you are told and speak when you are spoken to. But it is *your* diabetes and *your* body, and it is important that you take an active interest in what is happening to you. Asking questions is not troublemaking or being difficult. You must be involved in your diabetes and know what is going on, so that you can work with your advisers to keep as healthy as possible. They cannot guess what you are thinking. I must stress again, if you are worried about something, or fed up or confused, please ask; that is what we are there for.

The learning process

No one can learn even the basics of diabetes overnight. Taking command of your diabetes is a process that takes several weeks or months to learn and years to refine. It is important to learn to walk before you start running. This is not a beginner's book. If you are unsure about aspects of the basic knowledge I have assumed you know, do not be afraid to ask. The father of one of our diabetic patients is a teacher. He tells his son and his pupils: 'No question is ever silly if it has to be a question.' If you have got into a muddle with some aspect of your diabetes it is often helpful to go back to the beginning and work it out step by step. Sometimes when one is learning, or studying something, it helps to watch someone else going through the learning process and see the steps they have to take. Ben's story is of a young man just beginning to take command of his diabetes. Does any of it sound familiar to you? What advice would you give him from your experience of diabetes?

Ben's story

Ben is twenty-one years old and left school at sixteen to train in a technical drawing office. He had always enjoyed sports and continued this interest after he left school. Gradually he realized that he wanted to teach sports full time and applied for a physical education course. He was told that he would need more qualifications first, so he enrolled in another college for a year to obtain them.

He was working hard and everything was going well when he started to feel increasingly thirsty, had to keep leaving the room to pass urine and found that he was so tired that he could not manage his weight-lifting any more. He got thinner and felt awful. Three weeks after the onset of his symptoms he started vomiting, and was admitted to the hospital with early diabetic ketoacidosis. After a week of stabilization of glucose and fluid balance he was discharged on insulin injections and a diabetic diet.

I first met Ben in our Young Adult Diabetic Clinic a week after his discharge from the hospital. Initially he seemed uncertain and uncomfortable in the clinic, but gradually he started to talk. He said that he had gone straight back to college after his discharge from the hospital, but that he could not concentrate on his work. He was worried about the effect that this would have on his examination prospects during this precious year at college.

He was giving his own insulin injections and said he had no difficulties with this. He told me that he was measuring his blood and urine glucose levels four times a day.

He was bursting with questions. How was he going to manage his evening injections when he went out in the evening? Does insulin go off very fast if you do not keep it in the refrigerator? What about his weight-lifting? How could he work out regular meals and insulin when his lifestyle was very erratic, varying from sitting in lectures to very strenuous training? Why was he feeling so depressed?

A lot of questions, all muddled up. The thing that was worrying Ben most was his depression and inability to concentrate. We talked about how he felt when he learned that he had diabetes and that he would need insulin injections for the rest of his life. We discussed the possibility that one part of his mind could look at this logically and not be upset by it, but that deep down the rest of his mind needed time to adjust. We considered the effect sudden hospital admission has on everyone and that one needs time to convalesce after an acute illness like diabetic ketoacidosis. Impairment of concentration can be associated with depression and both can occur during fluctuations in glucose level and changes in body fluid and mineral balance. I asked if he had any special worries or fear about diabetes, but he said he had not. It was clear that we would need several sessions to talk about the subject and help Ben to come to terms with his diagnosis.

The next step was to see how Ben was coping with the mechanics of being diabetic. He was trying hard with the diet but was finding it difficult to cope with his large appetite with a limited dietary knowledge. He seemed to be living on wholewheat bread! I arranged for him to see the dietitian and reminded him that diet did not necessarily mean calorie restriction, but rather, attention to nutrition. I checked his insulin drawing up and injection technique and both were excellent. He also had good knowledge of when his insulins acted and for how long. What about testing? Ben's record was meticulously clear. We established that his urine glucose levels tallied with his blood tests, in other words that his renal threshold was normal. His blood glucose results showed high levels in the evenings, but were otherwise between 4 mmol/l (72 mg/dl) and 7 mmol/l (126 mg/dl) and he had had no hypoglycaemic attacks. I told him that there was no need to do both urine and blood glucose tests four times a day and suggested just using blood tests at present but, if he wished, substituting some urine tests if his fingers got sore.

Before talking about diet, insulin and glucose balance in more detail, I needed to know about his energy output. This naturally led to a discussion of his work at college and his sporting activities. We talked about planning for those activities and having regular meals; and coping with variable activities, such as the occasional afternoon swim or a night out with his friends. We discussed his resumption of evening training, which would almost certainly bring down his high evening glucose levels. I explained that diabetes was no deterrent to his planned career in sports education and he seemed very relieved. I think that secret worries about this may have been a major cause of his depression. We spent a considerable time discussing the details of his sporting activities and ways of adjusting his diet and insulin to allow him to perform at his best.

Thinking about Ben's energy output led to a discussion of the effect of diabetes on his social life. He was worried that his insulin would go off too fast for him to carry it with him when he was away from home in the evening. Again, I saw visible relief on his face when I told him that this was not the case. He had thought he would be restricted to home by the need for evening insulin injections. We talked about practical solutions to the problem.

Ben was also uneasy about what to tell his friends. It must be the truth, of course, but only when he felt ready, and then in a matter-of-fact way. Obviously, I suggested that his close friends should know so that they would be able to help him if he had a hypoglycaemic attack. I also said that Ben should tell his college tutors that he had become diabetic, so that they could arrange for extra study as he gradually felt better to help him make up for lost time. I offered to talk to them if Ben wanted me to do so.

He agreed that things did not look quite so black now. We arranged to meet in the clinic again soon. Gradually we shall work our way through all the relevant topics in this book. I shall also help him build up a plan for the care of his diabetes and for learning more about the condition and advances in treatment in the future. Some of these suggestions may also help you.

Join your local diabetic association

The addresses of the British, American, Australian and New Zealand Diabetic Associations are given at the back of this book. It is well worth joining your national association and its local branch. They produce magazines full of information not only of practical use, but also about recent research and new advances. The association may be able to help you with specific problems, such as advising on insurance or helping to find a particular piece of equipment. They run courses and vacations for people of all ages with diabetes. Some people say, 'Why should I join an association full of diabetics? I live in the non-diabetic world, I do not want to emphasize my condition.'

The point is that diabetics can do a lot to help each other and can provide the impetus for research into their condition, and help to raise money to fund it. You do not have to go to meetings unless you want to, but it is worth joining one of the associations just for the information service and magazines it provides.

Educate those around you

Life will be much easier if your family, friends and colleagues know that you have diabetes. It means that you can work out the problems of your diabetes in front of them if you have to, without being embarrassed.

You can also tell them what to do if you have a hypoglycaemic attack. If you are relaxed about it, they will be too. By showing them that diabetes does not interfere with your being an efficient employee, a good friend, a supermum, you are teaching them to be a little more receptive to the next diabetic person they meet.

Some people with diabetes are kind enough to help others who are in difficulties. Their help is especially important for those who have just been diagnosed diabetic. If they see that you are happy, fit and well, they will be much less frightened at the prospect of having diabetes for the rest of their lives. If you would like to do this, to offer your help to your local diabetic association or hospital, it will be greatly appreciated. A few centres run courses for diabetics to learn how to teach others about their condition.

Reminders

Here are some of the things you should check or have checked for you. Use these lists as a quick reference for maintaining good diabetic control.

Your lifestyle

1. Your diet should be high in fibre and low in saturated fats and sugary foods (refined carbohydrates), with no added salt. It should contain the right number of calories for you to achieve and remain at the ideal body weight for your height. Review your diet with a dietitian or nutritionist at least once a year.
2. Take regular exercise appropriately graded for your age and fitness level.
3. Do not smoke.
4. Drink alcohol in moderation only.
5. Get the amount of sleep and relaxation you need.

Your glucose balance

1. Test your blood glucose concentrations at least once a week, preferably once a day or more often. Check your measuring technique when you visit your diabetic adviser (I shall refer to a clinic visit from now on for simplicity), preferably against a venous laboratory glucose measurement.
2. Test your urine glucose concentrations, if you wish, at least once a week, preferably once a day or more often. Check your measuring technique at the clinic.
3. Your haemoglobin A_{1c} should be checked at every clinic visit (if these are more than a month apart).
4. Test your urine ketone concentrations if your glucose is high, or you feel ill or are pregnant.

Your drugs

Make sure you have the following:

1. Insulin, in date, enough for use and to cover breakages; stored correctly.
2. Your oral hypoglycaemic pills, in date, enough for use and to cover loss.
3. Pills for other conditions, in date, enough for use and to cover loss.

Your equipment

You should have:

1. Blood testing kit. Lancets, automatic pricker, platforms for pricker if needed. Blood testing strips, in date, enough; water bottle if needed; watch with second hand. Meter, correctly calibrated, with battery charged. Meter cleaned regularly as recommended by the manufacturer.
2. Urine testing kit. Tablets or strips, in date, enough; test tubes and droppers, clean, and not cracked.
3. Insulin injection kit. Syringes, disposable, enough and to spare, correct markings for your insulin strength; glass (if used) – two, sterile, not sticking or loose, not cracked; needles, disposable or reusable, enough and to spare. Penpump, correctly set, batteries charged; enough vials or syringes and to spare; enough tubing and needles and to spare; help telephone number day or night.
4. Diabetes travel pack ready for action (see Chapter 11).
5. Diabetic card with your current insulin dose, address and diabetic clinic written on it. Telephone number to contact diabetes adviser.
6. Diabetic diary.

Yourself

1. Feet: wash every night and dry carefully; treat injuries promptly. Your doctor should check your feet at least once a year.
2. Vision: report changes, for example, in reading the newspaper, seeing road signs. Eyes: full visual acuity check and examination with an ophthalmoscope after dilating drops by an expert, once a year; more often if you have retinopathy.
3. Blood pressure measurement every time you see a doctor.
4. Blood fats measurement, fasting, at least once every year; more often if raised.
5. Arteries: foot pulses checked by your doctor at least once a year.
6. Heart: electrocardiogram at least once for the over thirties, and if you have chest pains.

7. Kidneys: a urine protein test, infection screen, and blood creatinine level test at least once a year; more often if you have protein in your urine.
8. Sensation: your doctor should check for sensory changes (especially in your feet) once a year.
9. Injection sites: change them frequently and look at them every time you inject. Your doctor or nurse should check them every time you go to the clinic.

The above are one doctor's suggestions for a minimum diabetic care plan. Your diabetic adviser may have different views, so discuss them with him.

Remember: you control your diabetes – it does not control you.

Now go out and enjoy life to the full.

GLOSSARY

Acidosis Condition in which the blood is more acid than normal.
Adipose tissue Body fat.
Adrenal gland Gland found above the kidney which makes adrenaline and steroid hormones.
Adrenaline (American name **Epinephrine**) Flight, fright and fight hormone produced by the adrenal gland under stress.
Angina Chest pain caused by insufficient blood supply to heart muscle (a form of ischaemic heart disease). Also known as angina pectoris.
Angiogram X ray examination of an artery.
Ankle oedema Swelling of the ankles.
Aorta The largest artery in the body running from the heart through the chest and abdomen. The aorta carries blood from the heart for distribution into other arteries around the body.
Arteriopathy Abnormality of artery.
Atherosclerosis Hardening and furring up of the arteries.
Artery Vessel which carries blood from the heart to other parts of the body.
Arthropathy Abnormality of joint.
Autonomic nervous system Nerves controlling body functions such as heart beat, blood pressure and bowel movement.
Autonomic neuropathy Abnormality of the nerves controlling body functions.
Background retinopathy The common form of diabetic retinopathy with microaneurysms, dot and blot haemorrhages and exudates.
Balanitis Inflammation of the penis.
Bed sores Ulcers in the skin and sometimes into deeper tissues over pressure points in someone lying or sitting in the same position for a long time.
Beta blocker Drugs which reduce high blood pressure, steady the heart and prevent angina. All the names and in -olol, eg atenolol.
Biguanide A type of blood glucose lowering pill.
Bladder Usually means urinary bladder. Bag in the pelvis where the urine collects before urination.

Blood pressure   BP. Pressure at which blood circulates in the arteries.

Candida albicans   Another name for the thrush fungus.

Carbohydrate   CHO Sugary or starchy food which is digested in the gut to produce simple sugars like glucose. Carbohydrate foods include candy or sweets, cakes, biscuits, soda pop, bread, rice, pasta, oats, beans, lentils.

Cardiac   To do with the heart.

Cardiac enzymes   Chemicals released by damaged heart muscle.

Cardiac failure   Reduced functioning of the heart causing shortness of breath or ankle swelling.

Carotid artery   Artery which runs through the neck to supply the head and brain.

Carotid angiogram   X ray of dye passing up the carotid arteries into the brain arteries.

Cataract   Lens opacity.

Cells   The tiny building blocks from which the human body is made. Cell constituents are contained in a membrane.

Cerebral embolus   Clot from another part of the body which lodges in an artery supplying the brain.

Cerebral haemorrhage   Bleed into the brain.

Cerebral infarct   Death of brain tissue due to insufficient blood supply.

Cerebral thrombosis   Clot in an artery supplying the brain.

Cerebrovascular disease   Disease of the arteries supplying the brain.

Charcot joints   Damaged joints in areas of neuropathy (rare).

Cheiroarthropathy   Stiffening of the hands.

Chiropodist   Someone who prevents and treats foot disorders.

Chiropody   Treatment and prevention of foot disorders.

Cholesterol   A fat which circulates in the blood and is obtained from animal fats in food.

Computerized tomogram   CT scan. X Ray which can take multiple very detailed films from different angles. Commonly used to look at the brain but whole body CT scanners are also available.

Congestive cardiac failure   Impaired pumping of the right ventricle of the heart causing ankle swelling.

Conjunctivitis   Inflammation of the conjunctiva (white of the eye and inner eyelid).

Constipation   Infrequent and/or hard bowel motions.

Continuous ambulatory peritoneal dialysis   CAPD. A out-patient system of filtering wastes from the body of someone in kidney failure. Clean fluid is run into the abdominal cavity, takes up the waste substances and is run out again.

Continuous subcutaneous insulin infusion   CSII. A system for the constant pumping of insulin through a fine needle left under the skin all the time. Also known as an insulin pump.

Coronary artery   Artery which supplies the heart muscle.

Coronary thrombosis   Clot in an artery supplying heart muscle.

Creatinine   Chemical produced by breakdown of protein in the body and passed through the kidneys into the urine. A measure of kidney function.

Cystitis   Inflammation of the urinary bladder.

Diabetes mellitus   Condition in which the blood glucose concentration is above normal causing passage of large amounts (diabetes – a siphon) of sweet urine (mellitus – sweet like honey).

Diabetic amyotrophy   A form of diabetic nerve damage which causes weak muscles, usually in the legs.

Dialysis   Artificial filtration of fluid and waste products which would normally be excreted in the urine by the kidneys.

Diarrhoea   Frequent and/or loose bowel motions.

Diastolic blood pressure   Blood pressure between heart beats.

Diet   What you eat.

Dietitian   Someone who promotes a healthy diet and recommends dietary treatments.

Diuretic   Pill which increases urinary fluid loss. Diuretics are used to treat cardiac failure and most are also effective blood pressure lowering drugs.

Dot and blot haemorrhage   Tiny bleeds into the retina in diabetic retinopathy.

Dupuytren's contracture   Tightening of the ligaments in the palm of the hand or fingers.

Dysphasia   Difficulty in talking.

Dysuria   Pain or discomfort on passing urine.

Echocardiography   Examination of the heart using ultrasound waves from a probe run over the skin of the chest.

Electrocardiogram   ECG or EKG. Recording of the electrical activity of the heart muscle as it contracts and relaxes.

Electrolytes   Blood chemicals such as sodium and potassium.

Enzyme   Body chemical which facilitates other chemical processes.

Epinephrine   see adrenaline.

Essential hypertension   High blood pressure for which no specific cause can be found.

Exudate   Fatty deposit on the retina in retinopathy.

Fat   Greasy or oily substance. Fatty foods include butter, margarine, cheese, cooking oil, fried foods.

Femoral artery   The main artery supplying a leg. The femoral pulse can be felt in the groin.

Femoral arteriogram   X ray of dye injected into a femoral artery.

Fibre   Roughage in food. Found in beans, lentils, peas, bran, wholemeal flour, potatoes etc.

157

Fluoroscein angiogram   X ray of fluoroscein dye passing through the blood vessels in the eye.

Gastrointestinal   To do with the stomach and intestines.

Gastroenteritis   Inflammation or infection of the stomach and intestines.

Glaucoma   Raised pressure inside the eye.

Glomeruli   Tangles of tiny blood vessels in the kidneys from which urine filters into urinary drainage system.

Glucose   A simple sugar obtained from carbohydrates in food. Glucose circulates in the blood stream and is one of the body's main energy sources.

Glycaemia   Glucose in the blood.

Glycogen   The form in which glucose is stored in liver and muscles.

Glycosuria   Glucose in the urine.

Glycosylated haemoglobin   See haemoglobin A1.

Guar gum   A substance which slows the absorption of carbohydrate from the gut.

Gustatory sweating   Sweating while eating.

Haemodialysis   Artificial filtration of blood in someone with kidney failure.

Haemoglobin A1$_c$ Haemoglobin (the oxygen carrying chemical in the red blood cells) to which glucose has become attached. A long term measure of blood glucose concentration.

Haemorrhage   Bleed.

Heart   Muscular organ which pumps blood around the body.

Heart attack   General non-specific term for myocardial infarction or coronary thrombosis.

Hormone   A chemical made in one part of the body and acting in another part of the body.

Hyper-   High, above normal.

Hyperglycaemia   High blood glucose concentration (ie above normal).

Hypertension   High blood pressure.

Hypo-   Low, below normal.

Hypoglycaemia   Low blood glucose concentration (ie below normal).

Hypotension   Low blood pressure.

Hypothermia   Low body temperature.

Impotence   Difficulty in obtaining or maintaining a penile erection.

Infarction   Condition in which a body tissue dies from lack of blood supply – irreversible.

Insulin   A hormone produced in cells of the Islets of Langerhans in the pancreas. Essential for the entry of glucose into the body's cells.

Insulin dependent diabetes   IDD see Type I diabetes.

Insulin receptor   Site on the cell surface where insulin acts.

Intermittent claudication   The intermittent limping caused by insufficient blood supply to the leg muscles.

Intravenous pyelogram X ray of the kidneys showing the excretion of dye injected into a vein.

Ischaemia Condition in which a body tissue has insufficient blood supply – reversible.

Ischaemic heart disease An illness in which the blood supply to the heart muscle is insufficient

Islet cells Cells which produce insulin.

Islets of Langerhans Clusters of cells in the pancreas. One form of islet cells produces insulin.

Juvenile onset diabetes Diabetes starting in youth. This term implies a need for insulin treatment. Type I diabetes.

Ketoacidosis A state of severe insulin deficiency causing fat breakdown, ketone formation and acidification of the blood.

Ketones Fat breakdown products which smell of acetone or pear drops and make the blood acid.

Kilocalories Cals or kcals. A measure of energy, for example in food or used up in exercise.

Kilojoules Another measure of energy. One kilocalorie = 4.2 kilojoules.

Left ventricular failure Reduced functioning of the left pumping chamber of the heart causing fluid to build up in the lungs and shortness of breath.

Left ventricle Chamber of the heart which pumps oxygenated blood into the aorta.

Lens The part of the eye responsible for focussing (like the lens of a camera).

Lipid General name for fats found in the body.

Liver Large organ in upper right abdomen which acts as a energy store, chemical factory and detoxifying unit and produces bile.

Macroangiopathy Macrovascular disease.

Macrovascular disease Disease of large blood vessels such as those supplying the legs.

Macula Area of best vision in the eye.

Macular oedema Swelling of the macula.

Malaise Feeling vaguely unwell or uncomfortable.

Maturity onset diabetes Diabetes starting over the age of thirty. This term usually implies that the person is not completely insulin deficient, at least initially. Non-insulin dependent diabetes. Type II diabetes.

Metabolism The chemical processing of substances in the body.

Microalbuminuria The presence of tiny quantities of protein in the urine.

Microaneurysm Tony blow-out in the wall of a capillary in the retina of the eye.

Microangiopathy Microvascular disease.

Microvascular disease Disease of small blood vessels such as those supplying the eyes or kidney.

Moniliasis Thrush.

Myocardial infarction Death of heart muscle caused by lack of blood supply.

Myocardium Heart muscle.

Necrobiosis lipoidica diabeticorum Diabetic skin lesion (rare).

Nephropathy Abnormality of the kidney.

Nerve Cable carrying signals to or from the brain and spinal cord.

Neuroelectrophysiology Study of the way nerves work.

Neuropathy Abnormality of the nerves.

Nocturia Passing urine at night.

Non-insulin dependent diabetes NIDD Type of diabetes in which insulin treatment is not essential initially. See type II diabetes.

Nutritionist Someone who studies diets. Nutritionists may be dietitians and vice versa.

Obese Overweight, fat.

Obesity Condition of being overweight or fat.

Oedema Swelling.

Ophthalmoscope Magnifying torch with which the doctor looks into your eyes.

Oral Taken by mouth.

- pathy Disease or abnormality, eg neuropathy, retinopathy.

Palpitations Awareness of irregular or abnormally fast heart beat.

Pancreas Abdominal gland producing digestive enzymes, insulin and other hormones.

Paraesthesiae Pins and needles or tingling.

Peripheral nervous system Nerves supplying the skeletal muscles and body sensation such as touch, pain, temperature.

Peripheral neuropathy Abnormality of peripheral nerves eg those supplying arms or legs.

Peripheral vascular disease Abnormality of blood vessels supplying arms or legs.

Photocoagulation Light treatment of retinopathy.

Podiatrist Someone who prevents and treats foot disorders.

Podiatry Treatment and prevention of foot disorders.

Polydipsia Drinking large volumes of fluid.

Polyunsaturated fats Fats containing vegetable oils such as sunflower seed oil.

Polyuria Passing large volumes of urine frequently.

Postural hypotension Fall in blood pressure on standing.

Potassium Essential blood chemical.

Pressure sores See bedsores.

Protein   Dietary constituent required for body growth and repair.

Proteinuria   Protein in the urine.

Pyelonephritis   Kidney infection.

Pruritis vulvae   Itching of the vulva or perineum.

Receptor   Place on the cell wall with which a chemical or hormone links.

Renal   To do with the kidney.

Renal glycosuria   The presence of glucose in the urine because of an abnormally low renal threshold for glucose.

Renal threshold   Blood glucose concentration above which glucose overflows into the urine.

Retina   Light sensitive tissue at the back of the eye.

Retinopathy   Abnormality of the retina.

Right ventricle   Chamber of the heart which pumps the blood from the body into the lungs to be oxygenated.

Right ventricular failure   Reduced functioning of the right pumping chamber of the heart causing fluid to build up in the legs and ankle swelling.

Saturated fats   Animal fats such as those in dairy products, meat fat.

Sign   Something you can see, touch, smell or hear.

Sodium   Essential blood chemical.

Steroid hormone   A hormone produced by the adrenal gland.

Stroke   Abnormality of brain function (eg weakness of arm or leg) due to disease of the arteries supplying the brain or damage to the brain.

Subcutaneous   The fatty tissues under the skin.

Sulphonylurea   A form of blood glucose lowering pill.

Symptom   Something a person experiences.

Systolic blood pressure   Pumping pressure.

Testosterone   Male sex hormone.

Thrush   Candidiasis or moniliasis. Fungal infection caused by candida albicans fungus. Produces white creamy patches and intense itching and soreness.

Thrombosis   Clotting of blood.

Thrombus   A blood clot.

Transient ischaemic attack   TIA. Short lived stroke with full recovery within 24 hours.

Triglyceride   Form of fat which circulates in the blood stream.

Type I diabetes   Diabetes due to complete insulin deficiency for which treatment with insulin is essential. Lack of insulin leads to rapid illness and ketone production. Juvenile onset diabetes. Insulin dependent diabetes.

Type II diabetes   Diabetes due to inefficiency of insulin action or relative insulin deficiency which can usually be managed without insulin injections, at least initially. Ketone formation is less likely. Maturity onset diabetes. Non-insulin dependent diabetes.

Ulcer   Open sore.

Ultrasound scan   Scan of a part of the body using sound waves.

Uraemia   High blood urea concentration.

Urea   Blood chemical, waste substance excreted in urine.

Ureter   Tube from the kidney to the urinary bladder.

Urethra   Tube from the urinary bladder to the outside world.

Urinary incontinence   Unintentional leakage of urine.

Urinary retention   Retention of urine in the bladder because it cannot be passed.

Urinary tract infection   UTI. Infection in the urine drainage system.

Visual acuity   Sharpness of vision.

Vitreous   Clear jelly in the eye between the retina and the lens.

Vitreous haemorrhage   Bleed into the vitreous.

Useful addresses

UNITED KINGDOM

Action on Smoking and Health (ASH)
5–11 Mortimer Street
London W1N 7RH

Age Concern
Astral House
1268 London Road
Norbury
London SW16 4ER

British Diabetic Association
10 Queen Anne Street
London W1N 0BD

British Sports Association for the Disabled
The Mary Glen Haig Suite
34, St Osnaburgh Street
London
NW1 3ND

Cory Brothers (Erecaid)
4 Dollis Park
London N3 1HG

Disabled Living Foundation
380 Harrow Road
London W9

Health Education Authority
Mabledon Place
London WC1

Help the Aged
St James Walk
London EC1R 0BE

In Touch
BBC Publications
PO Box 234
London SW1

Keep Fit Association
16 Upper Woburn Place
London WC1H 0QG

Medic-Alert Foundation
12 Bridge Wharf
156 Caledonian Road
London N1 9UU

Medical Shop
Freepost
Woodstock
Oxon OX7 1BR

Optical Information Council
57A Old Woking Road
West Byfleet
Surrey KT14 6LF

Outward Bound Trust
Chestnut Field
Regent's Place
Rugby CV21 2PJ

Partially Sighted Society
Queens Road
Doncaster
South Yorkshire
DN1 2NX

Ramblers Association
1–5 Wandsworth Road
London SW8 2XX

Royal National Institute for the Blind
224 Great Portland Street
London W1N 6AA.

The Sports Council (Greater London and South East Region)
PO Box 480
Jubilee Stand
Crystal Palace National Sports Centre
Ledrington Road
London SE19 2BQ

Synergist (Correcaid)
Genesis Medical
115 Gloucester Road
London SW7 4ST

AUSTRALIA

Diabetes Association of SA Inc
157 Burbridge Road
Hilton
SA 5033

Diabetic Association of WA
48 Wickham Street
East Perth
WA 6004

Diabetes Australia
33 Ainslie Avenue
Canberra City
ACT 2600

Diabetes Australia
65 Davey Street
Hobart
Tas 7000

Diabetes Australia (NSW)
149 Pitt Road
Redfern
NSW

Diabetes Australia (Queensland)
124 Gerler Road
Hendra
QLD 4011

Diabetes Education and Assessment Centre
74 Herbert Street
St Leonards
NSW 2065

Diabetes Foundation (Vic)
100 Collins Street
Melbourne
Vic 3000

Diabetes Research Foundation of WA
Queen Elizabeth II Medical Centre
Hollywood
Perth
WA 6000

CANADA

The Canadian Diabetes Association
(National Office)
78 Bond Street
Toronto
Ontario M5B 2J8

UNITED STATES

American Diabetes Association
National Service Center
PO Box 25757
1660 Duke Street
Alexandria
VA 22314

Independent Living Aids Inc
1500 New Horizon Boulevard
Amityville
NY 11701

Juvenile Diabetes Foundation International
432 Park Avenue South
New York
NY 10016

National Association for the Visually Handicapped
22 West 21st
New York
NY 10010

National Diabetes Information Clearing House
Box NDIC
Bethesda
MD 20892

Index

Page numbers in *italics* refer to the illustrations

62, *116*; gangrene, 73;
  intermittent claudication, 60–1,
  115
liver, glycogen stores, 107
local associations, 151

macroangiopathy, 60–2
maculopathy, 137
marathon running, 110
Mason type diabetes, 87,
maturity onset diabetes, 31, 52–3,
  65, 87
maturity onset diabetes of youth
  (MODY), 52–3, 87
medical checks, 97
meetings, business, 103
menstruation, 74
meters, blood glucose monitoring,
  15–18, 90, 103, 153
microalbuminaria, 59
microaneurysm formation, 55
microangiopathy, 59, 60
mothers, diabetic, 93–4
motion sickness, 137–8
mountain expeditions, 129–32
mountain rescue, 128–9
mountain walking, 112–13
mountaineering, 122–4, *124*
muscles: beta-blockers and, 114;
  cramp, 111, 124, 131; glycogen
  stores, 107, 109

needles, disposable, 33
nerves: autonomic neuropathy, 58,
  80; neuropathy, 57–9, 63, 137
neuropathy, 57–9, 63, 137;
  autonomic, 58, 80, 143
night exercises, Outward Bound
  courses, 127
nitrates, 115
nocturnal hypoglycaemia, 51, 132
non-insulin-dependent diabetes, 24,
  genetics, 87, 88
noradrenaline, 127
norepinephrine, 127
Novopen, 35, 71, 103
numbness, hands and feet, 57–8,
  137

obesity, 53, 62
oral contraceptives, 83–4
oral hypoglycaemic drugs, 153;
  adjusting dose, 39–41; air travel,
  138; alcohol flushing, 104–5;
  during pregnancy, 90; glucose
  balance, 52–3; and
  hypoglycaemia, 43–4; on
  Outward Bound courses, 121;
  shift work, 101; and traveller's
  tummy, 143; types, 39–40; and
  variable work patterns, 102
orienteering, 127–8
Outward Bound courses, 118–33
Outward Bound Trust (OB), 118
overdoses, insulin, 75

pancreas, artificial, 35
penis, thrush, 60
Penject, 35
Penpump, 35
pens, injection techniques, 34–5, *34*
periods, 74
photocoagulation, 137
pork insulin, 27–9, 38
postural hypotension, 58
potassium, 49, 51, 62
pregnancy, 89–92, 152
pricking fingers, 16, *17*
progestogen, 83–4
puberty, 73–4
pumps, CSII *see* CSII pumps
pyelonephritis, 59–60

quinine, 111, 131

rail travel, 137
recovery position, 45, *45*
retina, diabetic retinopathy, 55–6,
  56, 57, 89, 137
reviews, school, 67–8
rhythm method, contraception, 81
rock climbing, 122–4, *124*
ropes courses, 127
rubella, 89
running, 110

safety: abseiling, 122–3; driving,

169

136–7; mountain expeditions, 129–32; Outward Bound courses, 120; rock climbing, 122, 123–4
salt, 62, 131
school, 65–9
school trips, 68–9
sea sickness, 137–8
sea travel, 137–8
self-destructive diabetics, 75–6
sexual intercourse, 79–80
sexual relations, 78–85
sheaths, contraception, 81–2, *83*
shift work, 98, *99–100*
ski bags, 122, *123*, 135
skiing, 112
skin, injection sites, 38
smoking, 61, 73, 89, 115, 152
snow blindness, 112
sodium, 62
spermicides, 81–2, *83*, 84
sports courses, 113
sprinting, 110
squash, 113
starvation ketosis, 50–1, 43
sterilization, 84
stomach upsets, 142–3
stress, 105–6, 137
strokes, 61, 83
sulphonylurea drugs, 39–40, 105
sunburn, 112
sweating, 131
swimming, 110–11, 121, 124–5
syringes, 33, 71

teachers, 66
team sports, 113–4
teenagers, 69–76, 118
tennis, 113
tests: blood glucose monitoring, 13–19, *17*, 22–3, 153; for ketones, 49, 51; urine glucose tests, *17*, 19–23, 152, 153

tetanus injections, 98
thiazide drugs, 62
thrombosis, 83
thrush, 60, 80
time zones, air travel, 138–42
tingling, hands and feet, 57, 59
travel, 134–44
travel insurance, 143
travel packs, 130, 132, 134–5, *135*, 136, 138, 153
travel sickness, 137–8
traveller's tummy, 142–3

unconsciousness, 45, *45*, *46*, 120, 128–9
universities, 76–7
urinary tract infections, 58, 59–60
urine: ketones, 49, 131–2; proteinuria, 59; urine glucose tests, *17*, 19–23, 152, 153

vacations, sports, 113
vasectomy, 84
vitamin deficiencies, 58
vomiting, 52, 142–3

walking, 115; mountain, 112–3, 129–32
water, drinking, 131
water sports, 110–11
weather, on holiday, 144
white-water canoeing, 126
winter mountain walking, 112–3
winter sports, 112–3
withdrawal method, contraception, 81
work, 96–106

x-rays, 138

zinc, allergies, 39

OTHER POSITIVE HEALTH GUIDES ON DIABETES

DIABETES BEYOND 40 by Dr Rowan Hillson

This book has been written specifically for people with diabetes who are in their forties or older. In detailed but simple terms the book covers:

- what diabetes is
- looking after *your* diabetes
- diet
- exercise and relaxation
- oral hypoglycaemics
- insulin
- blood glucose control
- complications and prevention
- self-help
- enjoying everyday life

Dr Rowan Hillson, Consultant Endocrinologist at Hillingdon Hospital, has produced a comprehensive, informative and positive guide to the particulars of this disease as they relate to the older diabetic.

ISBN 0 356 14850 5
Price **£6.99**

DIABETES – A YOUNG PERSON'S GUIDE by Dr Rowan Hillson

Learning to live with diabetes and enjoying life to the full is helped by knowing more about the condition. The book describes some young people's experiences and how their diabetes affected them.

Dr Rowan Hillson, Consultant Endocrinologist at Hillingdon Hospital, has written a practical and reassuring guide which covers:

- diagnosis, symptoms and treatment
- food, weight control and exercise
- relationships and sex
- school, college and university
- leaving home
- starting work
- holidays and travelling

ISBN 0 356 15415 7
Price (in UK only) **£5.99**

THE DIABETICS' COOKBOOK by Roberta Longstaff and Professor Jim Mann

From Professor Jim Mann, author of *The Diabetics' Diet Book*, and nutritionist Roberta Longstaff, comes this collection of over 180 delicious recipes which broadens the scope of modern diabetic cookery. Not only does it provide a wide range of wholesome everyday recipes, but also introduces:

- dinner and drinks party dishes
- children's meals
- food for festive occasions

This is a high-fibre, low-calorie eating programme that is healthy for everybody, whether or not they have diabetes.

ISBN 0 356 20565 7
Price **£7.99**

DIABETIC DELIGHTS by Jane Suthering and Sue Lousley

Jane Suthering, food stylist and cookery writer, combines originality with sugar-free ingredients to produce over 140 mouthwatering recipes. Nutritionist Sue Lousley explains how these tempting and healthy recipes can be successfully included in a balanced diet without diabetic control.

- recipes for biscuits, soufflés, fruit and sponge cakes, exotic fruit salads, flans, jellies, custards, ices and many more favourite family desserts
- useful information on natural and artificial sweeteners
- unique recipe coding system
- over 45 recipes illustrated in colour

These sugar-free, healthy recipes can be eaten by all the family – especially useful for slimmers on a calorie-controlled diet!

ISBN 0 356 20562 2
Price **£7.99**

PUBLISHED IN MARCH 1992, A BRAND NEW BOOK ON DIABETES

DIABETES: A NEW GUIDE by Dr Rowan Hillson

Consultant Endocrinologist at Hillingdon Hospital, Dr Rowan Hillson has written a new guide that assumes no previous knowledge or understanding of the subject. Although designed for the person whose diabetes is newly diagnosed, and their family and friends, there will also be much of interest, in the way of new ideas and information, to the experienced diabetic.

Illustrated throughout with case histories and helpful charts and diagrams, all information is related to whether someone is insulin-treated, tablet-treated or solely diet-treated, so the book is fully comprehensive in its coverage from first diagnosis to long-term self-health care.

ISBN 0 356 18769 1

Price **£7.99**

THE DIABETICS' DIET BOOK by Professor Jim Mann

This is the first book for diabetics and their dieticians that shows how to change to the new high-carbohydrate-and-fibre diet now being recommended by leading diabetic organisations around the world.

'The first easily available practical guide to healthy eating for diabetics.'

The Sunday Times

'High-fibre diet scores again – this time for diabetics.'

Daily Express

Full of imaginative recipes and beautifully illustrated.'

The Observer

ISBN 0 356 14475 5
Price **£3.95**

DIABETES AND PREGNANCY by Anna Knopfler

Pregnancy in diabetic women is a topic surrounded by a great deal of ignorance and many people still believe that insulin-dependent women rarely give birth to healthy babies. Author and diabetic mother Anna Knopfler, who set up the Diabetic Pregnancy Network, provides diabetic women with all the information they need on pregnancy and dispels all the myths.

Incorporating first-hand accounts, as well as advice from doctors, the book is a comprehensive guide from pre-conceptual care, through each stage of pregnancy, to post-natal health of the mother and baby. With photographs and illustrations, all aspects of diabetes care and pregnancy are examined with practical advice given.

ISBN 0 356 15189 1
Price **£5.99**

All Optima books are available at your bookshop or newsagent, or can be ordered from the following address:

Optima Books
Cash Sales Department
PO Box 11
Falmouth
Cornwall TR10 9EN

Alternatively you may fax your order to the above address. Fax number: 0326 76423

Payments can be made as follows: Cheque, postal order (payable to Little, Brown and Company) or by credit cards, Visa/Access. *Do not send cash or currency.*

UK customers, please send a cheque or postal order (no currency) and allow 80p for postage and packing for the first book plus 20p for each additional book up to a maximum charge of £2.00.

BFPO customers, please allow 80p for the first book plus 20p for each additional book.

Overseas customers, including Ireland, please allow £1.50 for postage and packing for the first book, £1.00 for the second book and 30p for each additional book.

NAME (Block letters) ....

ADDRESS ....

....

I enclose my remittance for _____

I wish to pay by Access/Visa Card

Number ☐☐☐☐☐☐☐☐☐☐☐☐☐☐☐☐

Card expiry date